HYSOMETRICS
A Hybrid program of weight training & Isometrics

Published by Urban Viking

(Urban Viking LTD, UK)

Copyright © 2023 by Kevin B. DiBacco

DISCLAIMER

No part of this publication may be reproduced in any form or by any means, including printing, scanning, photocopying, or otherwise without the prior written permission of the copyright holder. The author has attempted to present information that is as accurate and concrete as possible. The author is not a medical doctor and does not write in any medical capacity. All medical decisions should be made under the guidance and care of your primary physician. The author will not be held liable for any injury or loss that is incurred to the reader through the application of any of the information herein contained in this book. The author makes it clear that the medical field is fast evolving with newer studies being done continuously, therefore the information in this book is only a researched collaboration of accurate information at the time of writing. With the ever-changing nature of the subjects included, the author hopes that the reader will be able to appreciate the content that has been covered in this book. While all attempts have been made to verify each piece of information provided in this publication, the author assumes no responsibility for any error, omission, or contrary interpretation of the subject matter present in this book. Please note that any help or advice given hereof is not a substitution for licensed medical advice. The reader accepts responsibility in the use of any information and takes advice given in this book at their own risk. If the reader is under medication supervision or has had complications with health-related risks, consult your primary care physician as soon as possible before taking any advice given in this book.

"The information and advice contained in this book are based upon the research and the personal and professional experiences of the author. They are not intended as a substitute for consulting with a healthcare professional. The publisher and author are not responsible for any adverse effects or consequences resulting from the use of any of the suggestions, preparations, or procedures discussed in this book. All matters pertaining to your physical health should be supervised by a healthcare professional."

FOREWORD
PROFESSIONAL ENDORSEMENTS

Isometric strength training is one of the most underrated, and sometimes forgotten, strategies for building strength. Isometric conditioning of the muscles enjoys a great safety profile, generally with minimal risk for injury. Kevin has mastered the science of isometric conditioning, and has put together programs that safely, effectively build quality muscle.

Dr. Val Fiott
ACE-Certified Health Coach and Personal Trainer, Subject Matter Expert for the American Council on Exercise.
drval.perfectpersonaltraining.com

———————————————————————

I came across this wonderful book by Kevin. Isometric exercise has changed the way I work out, and it has helped me build up muscle without the wear and tear of traditional weight-lifting exercises. "Kevin has explained the exercise programs in simple words, and I would highly recommend this book to anyone who wants to know more about isometric training."

Dr. Fatima Tanveer, MBBS, M.D., ECFMG certified, Internal Medicine. MD Pakistan, Physician and International Medical Research Health, Medical & Lifestyle writer, South Asia.

Table of Contents

The MOTIVATION for this book:

This Entire workout program was the net result of finding a safe and effective way to rehab from two back-to-back hip replacement surgeries.

From 1979 to the present day, I was considered a gym rat. A guy that spent hours in the weight room getting stronger and bigger. My specialty was POWERLIFTING. I was never really a bodybuilder, although I trained MS. Connecticut and Mr. Teenage Florida back in the 1980's. My thing was to lift heavy. Being Strong was more important to me than looking like a bodybuilder. I would eventually compete in small New England push and pull contests with my friends to see how we would do. At my peak I was deadlifting six hundred pounds and bench pressing a max of five hundred and fifteen pounds. So, I was in the strong category for someone weighing only 245 lbs.

After twenty years of competitive powerlifting, my body began to break down. Multiple Knee Surgeries, Back surgeries, torn ligaments slowed me down in my forties. My love for lifting at the gym and the friends I made has really never left me.

In recent years, a severe back injury from work left me with nerve damage for life. Add the Knee surgeries with back surgeries and now my body has lost all its balance and symmetry. It was just a matter of time before Powerlifting and its injuries caught up to me.

Late in 2017, I noticed sharp pains shooting across my pelvis after snow blowing one day. After visiting my Orthopedic Surgeon, they discovered that both of my hips were 'narrowing' as they call it. Which basically means the space in the joint of your hip is closing causing devastating pain.

Again, with all my previous surgeries they surgeons were not going to guarantee that hip replacement would fix the pain. I was given a 50/50 chance.

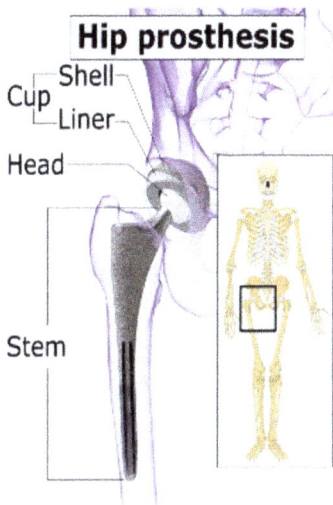

Hip prosthesis

Cup — Shell
— Liner

Head

Stem

Having nerve damage already, it was a crap shoot. I had not been in the gym for about six years because of my back. I researched new ways to train at home without doing any more damage to my back or knees. I had agreed to have one hip replaced at this point.

A professional wrestler friend of mine in Los Angeles sent me an eBook on Isometrics. Living in the wrestling world many of those guys have had multiple surgeries and must keep working. I knew about isometrics. We all did Isometrics as kids in gym class. I was in the Service where Isometrics was a daily way to train. The book he sent me was an in-depth program on isometrics exercises for each body part.

While limping around in severe pain, eating pain pills like candy, I decided to read the book. It was very inspiring. In fact, I asked my friend a zillion questions on how Isometrics can help you become strong. I was hooked.

This was the one way I could recapture my massive strength without having to limp around a gym.

I began a search for everything I could find on Isometric Training. Read medical research, University studies, doctors notes. Anything and everything I could find. That summer I purchased some dumbbells, Resistance bands and a workout bench.

With Hip Replacement surgery scheduled for October, I thought this would be the perfect time to drop some weight and get my body ready for recovering. At that time, I weighed 265 pounds. Far too heavy for someone not working out. I copied a few of the basic Isometric programs to learn the movements. It was incredibly hard. At this time, my right hip had totally 'crashed' meaning the space was gone and my bones were rubbing together. I had both back and knee surgeries, so I knew the pain. This was a shattering pain running down my legs, back and groin area.

So, I began Isometrics. Started slow. Trained twice a week. Tweaked my workouts. Tried different exercises, different combinations, different static hold times. I began to use my bands to do reps along with Isometric Static holds.

It was then that I found the secret. After three months of training, I developed this system. Combining Isometrics with Dynamic reps with bands and dumbbells. By summer's end I lost 30 pounds. I was getting much stronger and with a month left to surgery I was feeling good.

I went into surgery, in much better shape, mentally and physically. Recovery was NOT fun. The pain was still there, there was not much relief. After a couple of weeks, I noticed that I had pain in different areas. I told my doctors and they agreed that during the follow-up visit they would take a deeper look. Turns out that my left hip had narrowed in the time I was limping around all summer. The pain was coming from the other hip now! Surgery two was scheduled.

This time I had two months to get ready. I knew what to expect at least this time. I took my Isometric program to the next level. Each week I tried some new combination, new weights, exercises. I kept fine tuning my isometric workout, now called (HYSOMETRICS) a hybrid workout consisting of Isometrics, weightlifting, Aerobics & Body Weight exercises.

I kept a detailed log, and for the next six weeks I was able to pinpoint exactly what worked and what did not work at all! I dropped another fifteen pounds and went into surgery number two lighter and much stronger.

Another six weeks of recovery. This time I added in a stationary bike to rehab both hips. I went back into my notes and added a third day of Hysometric training. In three short months I lost another twenty pounds. I was twice as strong. The bike helped build my leg and hip muscles and I continued to dazzle the doctors who gave me a 50/50 chance that I may never get rid of the pain. I did. As of this writing, during the last follow-up visit my doctors were Amazed. They said they never had anyone recover and become stronger after double hip replacement surgery.

That brings me too today. I sit here with two years of trial-and-error notes. What worked, what did not work. What builds strength, what builds muscle? What burned more calories, what was aerobics? I took all those notes and decided to help someone else that may have to go through a similar experience. I started a blog called Iso Quick Strength. Shared some ideas then decided others can benefit from what I learned in the past twenty-eight months.

This is the result of what I learned to do to help me go from the Hospital bed to living life stronger and in far less pain. I hope that you can use some of these techniques. The one thing that I do know, is that they absolutely work! If done properly, given the time and attention you will be stronger, in better shape, more toned and mentally sharper than you have ever been.

Have fun!

The PRINCIPLES of the
HYSOMETRIC POWER PROGRAM

1. **Positive and Constant mental reminders (repeated aloud)**

2. **ALWAYS working outside the box:**

3. **NEVER Doing the same exercises or series the same way**

4. **Keeping a workout log to evaluate weekly**

5. **Eating healthy, limiting calories to your maximum**

6. **Consistent 3 day a week program**

7. **Inventing NEW exercises and testing them**

ISOMETRICS THE BEGINNING

Alexander Zass (1888 – 26 September 1962) was a Russian trainer. He was better known by his stage names, **The Amazing Samson**, **Iron Samson**, or simply **Samson**, Zass has been credited as the "first Russian champion in weightlifting in the pre-Revolutionary era".

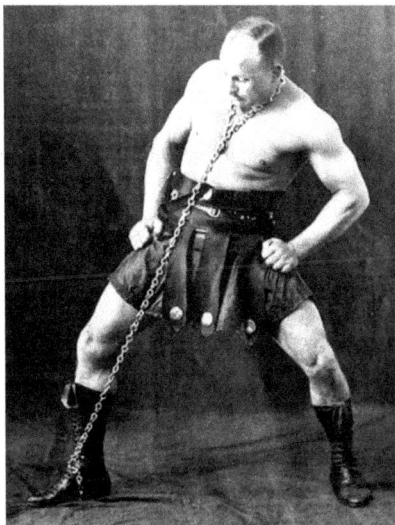

The Father of Isometrics- Alexander Zass

Biography

Zass was born in 1888 in Vilnius then part of the Russian Empire. While a young man, Zass' strength training included "bending green branches".

During WWI, Zass served in the Russian army, fighting against the Austrians. He was taken as a prisoner of war four times but managed to escape each time. As a prisoner, he pushed and pulled his cell bars as part of strength training, which was cited as an example and beginning of what we now know to be isometrics. At least one of his escapes involved him 'breaking chains and bending bars'. He went on to promote the use of isometric exercises.

Following the war, Zass joined a circus to perform feats of strength, touring internationally. It has been claimed that Zass was a spy and secret agent working for Russian military intelligence, using his circus traveling as cover. In 1926, his autobiography, *The Amazing Samson: as Told by Himself*, was published.

From the 1950s until his death, Zass lived in Hockley, Essex staying in a bungalow along with other former circus acts. He died in 1962; after a dawn funeral, he was buried in the parish church of St Peter & St Paul in Hockley, He was honored with a statue in a museum in Orenburg, Russia.

How Isometrics Work

Isometric exercise is great for building strength and muscle mass. It does 4 things by recruiting the most important motor units and increasing time under tension. Additionally, isometrics helps with the increase of the mind and muscle connection. I will touch on the mind/body connection a bit later. Improving your mind muscle connection increases the amount of muscle fiber recruited during lifting. When combined with increasing the time the muscle is under stress, it ends up in increased strength and muscle mass.

THE DEFINITION OF ISOMETRIC EXERCISE

Physical exertion may be a type of exercise involving the static contraction of a muscle with non-visible movement within the angle of the joint. "isometric" combines the Greek words "Isos" (equal) and "metria" (measuring), which means exercises the length of the muscle and therefore the angle of the joint do not change, though contraction strength could also be varied. This can contrast with isotonic contractions, within which the contraction strength does not change, though the muscle length and joint angle do. The three main sorts of exercise are isometric presses, pulls, and holds. They will be included in an extraordinarily intense training regime to boost the body's ability to use power from a static position or, within the case of isometric holds, improve the body's ability to take care of a foothold for a period of your time. Considered as an action, isometric presses are of fundamental importance to the body's ability to organize itself to perform immediately subsequent power movements. Such preparation is additionally called isometric preload.

WHAT ARE ISOMETRICS ?

Isometrics are exercises where your joints do not move. Normally during exercise, you move

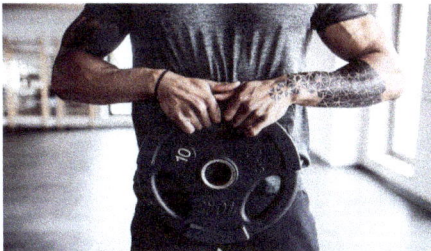

your joints through a full or partial range of motion. Think of the pull up, for example.

You start off hanging from a bar and slowly raise yourself up until Your chin is above the bar. In isometric exercises you stay in one spot.

There are 3 diverse types of isometrics:

Yielding

This type of isometric requires a force to be pushed against your muscle. A good example of this type of isometric is when you place your hands together and push as hard as you can. Your hands and arms do not go anywhere but you fatigue the muscle.

Overcoming

Overcoming isometrics are exercises where you push against an immovable force. A good example of this is pushing against a wall. When you push against a wall every muscle you have becomes engaged. The key to this style of isometric is to push with all your might. Give it everything you have and go until you are completely fatigued.

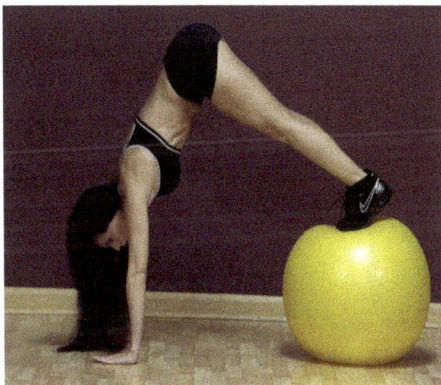

Static Tension.

In this type of isometric, you tighten the muscle but there is no movement or force against it. You are simply tightening the muscles. Like Posing a muscle.

2 KEY ELEMENTS TO PERFORMING ISOMETRICS

When engaging in these exercises, it is essential to focus on two key aspects:

1) Breath control: Pay close attention to your breathing patterns throughout the routine. There are three distinct phases of breathing during each isometric contraction.

Begin by inhaling deeply through your nose for a duration of 3 to 4 seconds. As you do this, gradually build tension in the targeted muscles. By the time you finish inhaling, the muscles you are working on should be under maximum tension.

Once your muscles reach peak contraction, proceed to exhale in a controlled manner through your mouth for 7 to 12 seconds. You can achieve this by creating a "sssssssss" sound, either through clenched teeth or pursed lips. Correct execution of the exhale should resemble the hissing of a snake or the gradual release of air from a tire. It is crucial to maintain maximum tension in the isometric contraction throughout the exhale.

To release the tension, slowly inhale through your nose again for a duration of 3 to 4 seconds. As you do so, gradually relax your muscles. By the time you complete the 4-second inhalation, your muscles should be fully relaxed.

2) Mental focus: Contrary to common belief, the ability to contract your muscles with

greater intensity and efficiency lies not within the muscles themselves, but within your mind. Your brain serves as the control center for your muscles. Therefore, it is imperative to direct your thoughts towards the muscles being worked on and execute each contraction with unwavering focus and intensity. For instance, if you are performing an isometric contraction on your biceps, envision the blood surging into the muscle and visualize its growth, strength, and enhanced definition. This mental approach is crucial to achieving optimal results.

BEGINNING OF ISOMETRICS

Let us begin with what the word isometric means. Merriam Webster online dictionary, has the definition as associated with fitness is an adjective meaning anything "of, referring to, involving, or being contraction (as in isometrics) against resistance, without significant shortening of muscle fibers, and with marked increase in muscular tone."

According to one study, physical exertion is defined as "exercise without motion or because they try to move an immovable object. The term isometric contraction comes from the fact that in isometric exercise there is no change within the length of the muscle. Iso means the same, metric means length. Although no work is finished, near maximum effort is extended." There are differing reports on the etymology of the word. Webster's claims that the primary known use of the word, on equality in measure, was in 1855. Based on another account, isometrics was first utilized in "1838, literally [to mean] "of the identical measure," from iso- "the same, equal" + -metric. The components are Greek: isos "equal, identical" + metron "a measure." Originally a technique of using perspective in drawing; later in relevance crystals. Most agree that the word isometric originated from the Greek word isos, which implies "the same," and metron which implies "size."

"Thus, isometric contraction means tensing the muscle without the muscle itself changing its length."

In the ancient Asia, exercising dates back 5000 years. Ancient martial artists and yogis created postures to honor deities of their respective cultures. There's evidence of self-defense forms dating to 3000 BC in countries like India, Pakistan, and Nepal. "What is thought is that martial arts began within the ancient cultures of Asia, including China, India, and Japan. In both China and India, artifacts from 2,000 to 4,000 years old are found with paintings of individuals striking possible martial arts poses. Buddhist monks created a "flow" of 12 self-resistance, or isometric exercises which were introduced to monks in China within the twelfth century.

30

Interpretations and variations of this series of postures have been practiced now for hundreds of years by martial artists across the world. Martial artists today still use the isometric practice of flowing from one fighting stance to a different in an exercise sequence. "The stillness in stillness isn't the important stillness; only there's stillness in movement does the universal rhythm manifest." Bruce Lee

Yoga is another original variety of physical exertion. It was first developed in ancient India. Yoga also dates to approximately 3000 BC supported stone carvings of a few of the primary yoga postures found within the Indus Valley. Yoga is equally accountable for the event of isometrics into the exercise form we all know today. The "flow" of exercise postures is recognized and related to the practice of yoga. Isometrics is an ancient style of exercise, for sure. Many modern styles of exercise methods have developed recently including hot yoga, Pilates with the employment of gravity alone. Isometrics needs no equipment. As in martial arts and yoga, only the employment of your body and gravity is needed. In some instances, basic tools like bands and suspension straps can enhance the performance of contemporary physical exertion. Isometric training is sweet for muscle toning and strength gains and there is zero impact to the structure of the body. Central Washington University research indicates that "isometric and isotonic exercises were the same in producing strength increases.

In 1953 two young German physicians by the name of Müller and Hettinger researched isometrics. They found that the leg of a frog attached to an unmovable object grew stronger than the opposite leg which was attached to a moveable weight. So, within the early 1960's isometrics suddenly appeared everywhere! Isometric exercises were adapted by high school athletic programs, little isometric workout books might be found at grocery check-out stands, and isometric exercises appeared on the backs of cereal boxes. The fad quickly came and slipped with bouffant hairdos and call box stuffing. The rationale for the isometrics craze disappeared as quickly as it had appeared, because the final public discarded isometrics when it had been discovered that nobody may be transformed into a gargantuan overnight. As is that the case in any physical development program, time, effort, and fortitude are essential ingredients. So, why isn't self-resistance exercise widely used or maybe widely known today? It is because exercise equipment is so readily available and aggressively marketed. You cannot watch tv without seeing another new device to tone your tummy that could be yours in 3 easy payments by just calling a toll-free number, with operators standing by to require your order. Quality gyms with state-of-the-art equipment are located on every other corner throughout the world. Discount stores are equipped with home gym and other fitness items. With just a MasterCard and a click of a button, a complete system can be delivered to your doorstep within a week.

BENEFITS OF ISOMETRICS

Isometrics are defined as **static** (rather than **dynamic**) exercises during which neither the muscle length nor the joint angle changes. Any exercise in which you contract a bunch of muscles and sustain that contraction for a given amount of your time, without moving at the joints, essentially would be considered physical exercise. For example, a classic biceps curl is taken into account as a dynamic exercise because jointly pulls the burden up toward the shoulder, the bicep muscle is shortened on the concentric contraction and so is lengthened because the weight is released and lowered backtrack on the eccentric contraction. In contrast, when one holds a plank position, the muscles of the rear, abdomen, and shoulders are all contracted, but they are held in this contraction for a considerable amount of your time with no change within the length of the muscles. A plank could be a static exercise and thus considered an isometric. If you have ever practiced Yoga, Pilates, or Barre, then you are already aware of isometric contractions, as many of the poses and exercises performed in these formats involve various varieties of isometrics. Isometric muscle contractions often challenge one's balance, which brings me to my next point: the numerous health benefits that isometrics provide. Improving one's balance and coordination is particularly important for the aging population pretty much as good balance helps in preventing injury from falls. Other health benefits that may be gained by incorporating isometrics into your fitness programs include:

- **Increases overall strength.**
- **Builds bone density.**
- **May help lower blood pressure**
- **Low impact exercises**
- **No need for special equipment**

Since isometric exercises are low impact, those recovering from shoulder and knee injuries can still partake (with caution, of course). One other additional benefit is that you may practice isometrics anywhere! Isometrics should be done on a weekly basis to reap the complete benefits. If not already an element of your fitness routine, it is recommended that isometrics be included in a very well-balanced program that might include strength training, cardiovascular and suppleness exercises. After all, it's all about finding balance, right?

#1 They are Safe.

This is the rationale we use so often in therapy following surgery (think complex body part repair). Often in these cases, the patient has a range of motion restrictions from the surgery. We wish to begin strengthening the muscles immediately, but we are not allowed to maneuver the joint. What can we do? Isometrics! The same principle will be applied to semi healthy folks understanding in their home gyms. If you have a known shoulder or knee problem, some exercises could also be painful. With the utilization of isometrics, you will be able to find a comfortable position and hold it for a given time to figure the muscle without pain. Isometric wall squats are an excellent example. Standard squats give people lots of knee issues. Whether it is because of incorrect form or patellar gliding issues, the results are the same- pain. Holding a wall squat isometrically in an exceedingly position allows you to figure your quads and glutes safely without having to be limited by discomfort.

#2 No Equipment Necessary.

There are times when you will have limited access to equipment. And then times like we are going through now with when Covid 19 hit, where gyms and fitness centers are closed. You will not have any equipment at all! That is ok. Isometrics are often done with zero equipment; all you would need is your body. But are there really enough bodyweight isometric exercises you can perform to form a workout out of them?

Yes!? Isometric wall squat (wall sit) Isometric push up, Plank Side plank Isometric bridge, Isometric lunge, Downward-facing dog, these are just some samples of isometric exercises you'll do without equipment. you will also notice that these moves don't require much floor space either- helpful if you've got limited room for your workouts. If you're into yoga, lots of these moves and postures are isometric exercises still.

#3 Can Improve Strength.

If you are using some equipment, like dumbbells or resistance bands, you'll be able to take your isometric exercises to a fully new level. Bodyweight exercises are great, but with some external resistance you'll be able to turn any exercise into an isometric move. You'll also see more impressive strength gains by using resistance together with your isometric moves. Research has shown that isometric moves can increase the strength at that specific joint angle. For instance, if you're holding an isometric bicep curl at 90 deg of elbow flex, the biceps will primarily become stronger at that 90 deg angle. there'll likely be some spill over within the few deg around that joint position. But who says you'll be able to only do isometrics at one joint position?!? How about holding isometric exercises at distinct positions to realize strength through a bigger range of motion? Sounds good to me. Using that very same bicep curl example, you may hold the position at 60 deg, 90 deg, and 120 deg.

Here are a few more exercises I think this strategy would work well with. Try them and see what you think:

- **Shoulder fly's**
- **Chest press**
- **Shoulder press**
- **Skull crushers**
- **Pec fly's**
- **Lat pulldown (resistance bands)**

You can also combine dynamic exercise with isometric holds. This is why this book is called HYSOMETRICS. The combination of dynamic exercises with Isometrics. Knock out a few dumbbell curls and then hold one rep isometrically.

40

#4 Improve Flexibility.

Isometric exercises may also be done to improve flexibility while you're improving strength. A downward-facing dog is one among the more famous yoga poses and it's accustomed to improving flexibility and strength at the same time. For those of you unfamiliar, it's kind of like holding a plank and a hamstring stretch at the identical time. You're visiting and really feel it on your shoulders. But it's also an excellent thanks to improve the flexibility in your hamstrings and calves. There are a large number of other yoga (and Pilates) positions that are designed to enhance strength and suppleness at the identical time. plenty of use tend to neglect stretching because, well, it isn't much fun to try to do. But isometric exercises can give us a more engaging thanks to staying loose and reducing our chance of injury.

#5 Can Lower Blood Pressure.

According to the American Heart Association. A 2013 study suggested that 4 weeks of isometric hand exercises lowered participants' blood pressure level by a mean of 10%. It was found that hand exercises were able to effectively lower force per unit area pressure levels, imagine what full body isometrics could do. We all know that cardiovascular exercise, like walking or riding a motorbike, could be an effective way to lower your vital sign. Now you'll take a step farther and add some isometric moves to your routine.

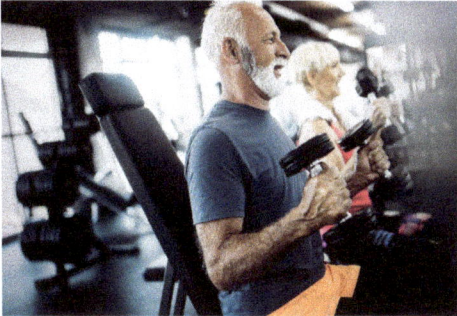

WHAT THE EXPERTS SAY ABOUT ISOMETRICS.

1. "Isometric resistance training lowers Systolic Blood Pressure, Diastolic Blood Pressure, and mean arterial pressure. The magnitude of effect is larger than that previously reported in dynamic aerobic or resistance training. Our data suggest that this form of training has the potential to produce significant and clinically meaningful blood

pressure reductions and could serve as an adjunctive exercise modality."

The Journal of the American Heart Association
2. "while there is direct evidence of an association between neck isometric training or strength and injury risk. A retrospective analysis of professional rugby union players revealed that isometric training reduced match-related cervical spine injuries and a prospective study found that greater overall isometric neck strength reduced concussion risk in high school athletes."

Sports Med
3. "This study suggests that greater isometric muscle strength in youth is associated with lower levels of cardiovascular risk factors in young adulthood independent of fitness, adiposity and other confounding factors."

The British Journal of Sports Medicine

4. "Older adults experienced similar reductions in pain following several different intensities and durations of isometric contractions.

American College of Sports Medicine
5. "Isometric cervical muscle strength mitigates head impact severity."

British Journal of Sports Medicine
6. "Isometric stabilization exercises reduce pain and enhance vitality as dimensions of Health-Related Quality of Life among women with chronic low back pain with such effects lasting for at least nine months."

Journal of Physical Health and Activity
7. "Isometric exercise is a fundamental component of both nonoperative and postoperative rehabilitation of shoulder instability."

Current Orthopedic Practice
8. "Data from a small number of isometric resistance training studies suggest this form of training has the potential for the largest reductions in Systolic Blood Pressure."

Journal of the American Heart Association
9. "Isometric strength training can have beneficial effects on performance during endurance events."

European Journal of Applied Physiology
10. "Isometric exercises not only prevent reduction of bone density but may also increase the mineral density of the injured bone."

Journal of the Facility of Medicine
11. "Early introduction of isometric exercise is a relevant choice in cases of patients with sciatica caused by disc herniation."

Isokinetic and Exercise Science

12. "Following musculoskeletal pathology, where a disorder of muscle onset timing has been identified, practitioners should consider the use of isolated (isometric) muscle training to restore the timing of muscle onset."

Physical Therapy in Sport

13. "Study revealed that localized isometric exercises have been effective in reducing the fat percentage."

Annals of Biological Research

14. "This data also suggests that increases in "isometric" strength may be associated with better hitting performance."

Chinese Journal of Sports Biomechanics
15. "These findings suggest that isometric training may be an important addition to ACL injury prevention programs."

Journal of Electromyography and Kinesiology
16. "Maximum isometric strength also is likely to have a strong role in weightlifting performance."

The Journal of Sports Medicine and Physical Fitness
17. "Besides blood pressure, isometric exercise is associated with other beneficial effects consisting of an increase in muscle bulk, upper and lower body strength, increases in bone density, and a decrease in bone fractures. These changes are extremely beneficial to older patients by making them more mobile and increasing their quality of life."

The Journal of Clinical Hypertension

18. "In fact, using isometric exercise for 6 minutes would be the equivalent muscle work of 30 to 35 minutes of gym work on commercial weightlifting equipment."

Journal of Applied Research

19. "Stretching and aerobic exercising alone proved to be a much less effective form of training than isometric strength training."

Journal of the American Medical Association

20. "The weight loss for some subjects in the first 2 weeks was as high as 8.4 kg while after 4 weeks (of isometric exercise). Some subjects lost as much as 10.1 kg in body weight."

The Journal of Applied Research

21. "In male and female athletes across the age spectrum, greater "isometric" neck strength and anticipatory cervical muscle activation ("bracing for impact") can reduce

the magnitude of the head's kinematic response."

The American Journal of Sports Medicine
22. "The results indicate that isometric exercise increased femoral bone blood flow from rest to low intensity exercise, but blood flow did not increase further with increasing intensity."

American Society for Bone and Mineral Research
23. "The results suggest that explosive force production during isometric squats was associated with athletic performance. Specifically, sprint performance was most strongly related to the proportion of maximal force achieved in the first phase of explosive-isometric squats, whilst jump height was most strongly related to absolute force in the later phase of the explosive-isometric squats."

Journal of Sports Sciences

24. "Explosive isometric training has been shown here to provide similar benefits to that of plyometric training with respect to the measured variables, but with reduced impact forces, and would therefore provide a useful adjunct for athletic training programs."

Journal of Strength and Conditioning Research

25. "The possibility of different energy costs is suggested by the fact that the metabolic changes resulting from a 30sec isometric contraction of the quadriceps are similar to those of a 30sec maximal sprint. During an isometric contraction, the muscle is continually active but when sprinting the quadriceps muscle is used only for a limited period during each stride, so the total duration of the muscle contraction during a 30 sec sprint can only be a fraction of the overall duration of the exercise."

Journal of Physiology

26. "In this group of patients we were able to show that guided isometric training of the paravertebral muscles can be safely practiced in palliative patients with stable bone metastases of the vertebral column, improving their pain score and mobility."

DON'T HOLD YOUR BREATH

One of the most important things to do in isometric moves is breathe. Isometric exercises require lots of oxygen and if you're holding your breath, you'll always plateau at round the 10 second mark. When I trained at the local gym, I'd see guys doing sets without breathing. Their faces would expand red, and they would sit around after just to catch their breath. Holding your breath when doing total body exercises goes to knock you out and if you're really pushing yourself, you may pass out - not good times! Isometric Breathing When doing isometric exercises, you'll struggle to require deep breaths in and out, and you shouldn't. If you are trying to breathe too deeply, you'll find yourself slipping out of the movement and doubtless collapsing on the ground.

Keeping your breathing shallow will enable you to stay your trunk tight because you're stuffed with air, you're always pulling oxygen into your blood, and you'll hold on for longer. Air cycles around your nose and mouth but it'll create movement around your lungs too. You may continuously move air in and out of your lungs without lots of effort because you'll keep your muscles tight.

Can Lower Pressure According to the American Heart Association, isometrics may help with lowering your pressure level. A 2013 study suggested that 4 weeks of isometric hand exercises lowered participants' force per unit area by a median of 10%. It seems amazing that hand exercises were ready to effectively lower force per unit area, imagine what full body isometrics could do. We all know that cardiovascular exercise, like walking or riding a motorbike, may be a clever way to lower your pressure level. Now you'll take a step farther and add some isometric moves to your routine.

How to:

- **Start with a nice big breath as you get into the hold, starting with full lungs will help keep them full**
- **As your whole body tightens, start to take shallow breaths through your nose and mouth.**
- **When your body starts trembling you will notice your breath cycling to that rhythm**

- **Bringing the air into your nose and mouth, combined with your body movement allows for little diaphragm movement, instead you are cycling air in and around your lungs continuously.**

NERVE POWER

Nerve power are some things the old-time strongmen talked about. After they said it they really meant the identical thing as many of the eastern philosophies mean after they speak about "Chi." It's a mix of the particular nerves that run through your muscles and make things happen when your mind tells the body to maneuver and also the subtle electrical current that flows round the whole body that truly makes those nerves function. Isometrics are proven to be one of the best ways to show your nerves or bring them up to their highest potential and thus bring your muscle's ability to contract up to its greatest strength. After you train you not only build your body strength, your tendons, ligaments and muscles, but also your nerve power. So, when you're trained all around from all angles you train your nerves and everyone their crossing routes and therefore the more angles you train the more developed your nerve highways are and therefore the better your endurance is all around. Since fiber recruitment is one in all the key neural factors affecting strength, frequent isometric training can program your system to be more efficient at recruiting more fibers. Once that's done, you may become stronger in your regular lifting exercises without adding muscle mass. One of the foremost important benefits of isometric action training is that it's the shape of contraction that facilitates the best muscular activation. By increasing activation, the amount of motor units that are wont to innervate and contract a vegetative cell are increased.

Research in 2003 exploring this idea has shown that maximal isometric training on the average, recruits approximately 5% more muscle fibers compared to maximal eccentric or concentric actions. This idea is supported by an oversized body of literature. Long term, the increased neural drive (the connection of the motor unit to the muscle) could positively enhance potential for strength gains.

Regarding the myelination process: in our bodies, electrical signals travel from one neuron within the body to a different (for example, from one neuron body to a muscle) on axons. The speed at which these electrical signals travel relies upon the extent at which the axon is coated with myelin. Myelin quickens the transmission of those electrical signals to the muscles by insulating the axon and reducing loss in electrical charge (higher the charge the larger the potential for the action). The target of myelination is to extend the nervous systems efficiency by improving the speed at which signals are sent and limiting energy loss. The purpose of implementing a phase dedicated strictly to myelination is to boost motor unit recruitment, which is able to improve activation of the muscle needed to perform the specified movement, while, at the identical time, deactivating the fibers that work against the specified outcome of the exercise. It's simply teaching the brain which motor units to fire to supply the specified movement. In your workout, it'll help develop motor skills that recruit large muscle groups for multi-joint movements. Developing these multi-joint movements or "big lifts" (squat, deadlift, bench press, etc.) within the off-season will transfer to stronger, faster, and more powerful athletes on the sphere during competition.

SIGNALING THE BRAIN

The myelination process: in our bodies, electrical signals travel from one neuron within the body to a different (for example, from one

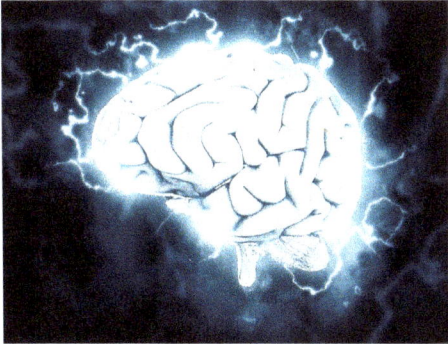

vegetative cell body to a muscle) on axons. The speed at which these electrical signals travel relies upon the amount at which the axon is coated with myelin. Myelin quickens the transmission of those electrical signals to the muscles by insulating the axon and reducing loss in electrical charge (higher the charge the larger the potential for the action). The target of myelination is to extend the nervous system's efficiency by improving the speed at which signals are sent and limiting energy loss. The Role of Isometrics helps to enhance the myelination process and to boost motor unit recruitment. This will improve activation of the muscle needed to perform the specified movement.

It's simply teaching the brain which motor units to fire to supply the specified movement. within the weight room, it'll help develop gross motor skills that recruit large muscle groups for multi-joint movements. Developing these multi-joint movements or "big lifts" (squat, deadlift, bench press, etc.) within the off-season will transfer to stronger, faster, and more powerful athletes. Overcoming Isometrics One of the crucial ways to program a myelination phase is through using Overcoming Isometrics (OI).

An OI is different from your typical isometric. OI exercises involve pushing or pulling against an immovable resistance or object. Using a rope or chain to pull against a tree or try to lift a truck. During the exercise, there'll be no external movement; however, the intent is to add maximum resistance. The muscle does not know if you are trying to curl 50 pounds or an SUV. All it knows is that it has to call in all of its resources to help attempt the lift.

An example would be pressing or pulling a bar against pins on a rack. There are many reasons why OI's are preferred to yielding isometrics during a myelination phase. I can tell you firsthand. Overcoming Isometrics builds Super Strength. The brain doesn't know how much you are trying to lift, it knows that you want to lift it so it's all hands-on deck. That means your brain is calling in every muscle to help.

During a study, it was found that in maximal OI muscle actions, there are higher levels of muscle activation **(95.2 percent)** than during maximal eccentric negative move **(88.3 percent)** and maximal concentric (89.7 percent) muscle actions. These findings state that a personal can recruit nearly all motor units during a maximal isometric contraction only, which improves neural drive and greatly increases their peak potential for strength and power.

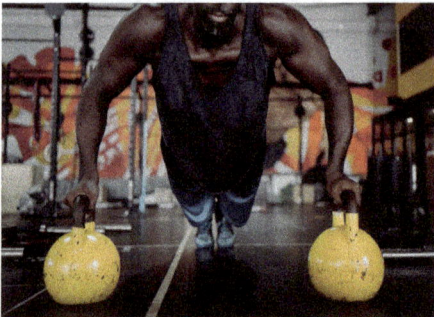

PURE STRENGTH

Physical strength might stem as much from exercising the nervous system as the muscles it controls. The findings could explain why those who lift heavier weights enjoy greater strength gains than low-load lifters despite similar growth in muscle mass.

I read a recent study from the University of Nebraska-Lincoln that has given new meaning to the concept of brain power by suggesting that physical strength might stem as much from exercising the nervous system as the muscles it controls.

Over the past few years, researchers have found evidence that lifting more repetitions of lighter weight can build muscle mass just as well as fewer reps of heavier weight. Even so, those who train with heavier weight still see greater gains in strength than those who lift lighter loads. Thus, making a 100% Isometric Contraction the ultimate strength builder.

Their study suggests that high-load training better conditions the nervous system to transmit electrical signals from the brain to muscles, increasing the force those muscles can produce to a greater extent than does low-load training.

Muscles contract when they receive electrical signals that originate in the brain's neuron-rich motor cortex. Those signals descend from the cortex to the spinal tract, speeding through the spine while jumping to other motor neurons that then excite muscle fibers.

Studies found evidence that the nervous system activates more of those motor neurons -- or excites them more frequently -- when subjected to high-load training. That increased excitation could account for the greater strength gains despite comparable growth in muscle mass.

"If you're trying to increase strength -- whether you're a weekend warrior, a gym rat or an athlete -- training with high loads is going to result in greater strength adaptations.

When adjusting for baseline scores, the researchers found that the voluntary activation of the low-load group increased from **90.07 to 90.22** percent -- 0.15 percent -- over a three-week span. The high-load group saw their voluntary activation jump from 90.94 to 93.29 percent, a rise of 2.35 percent.

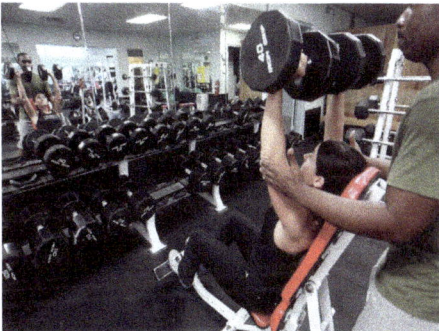

"During a maximal contraction, it would be advantageous if we are activating more motor units," The result of that should be greater voluntary force production -- an increase in strength.

That my friends is **EXACTLY what Isometrics does!**

KEY POINTS

Motor Neurons

Motor neurons are nerve cells that originate in the central nervous system and end at the muscle fibers in the neuromuscular junction. Signals sent from the brain run along the motor neuron to the muscle fiber to produce movements, or muscular contractions. When trying new exercises, an athlete's brain must send signals along motor neurons to the correct muscle fibers in order to contract.

When athletes lift heavier weights, the frequency of motor neurons firing increases and the number of muscle fibers contracting increases. Ultimately, the growth in motor neurons and muscle fibers builds muscle mass in athletes.

Muscle Memory

Muscle memory, also known as neuromuscular facilitation, is the process by which muscles become familiar with certain motor skills. Furthermore, when signals from the brain are sent to the muscle, a pathway becomes established, and this process becomes semi-automatic. Once this happens, athletes won't need to concentrate intensely to create the desired movement. It is likely that the muscle tissue will also develop long-lasting changes (i.e., increases in fiber size and changes in fiber composition).

Strength Training

Functional strength training helps athletes develop muscle memory so that they can quickly access their movement patterns during performance. The neuromuscular system goes through a cycle when developing strength: teach the brain to fire correct muscles to contract with a new movement, add resistance, recruit more muscle fibers to oppose the resistance, build strength and adapt to the resistance, increase the complexity or resistance, and repeat.

Additionally, performing strength exercises when the body is fatigued will teach the brain to recruit muscles when it normally does not. This adaptation is useful at the end of a race, game or event, when an athlete's strength normally begins to wane.

Jennifer Reed MD, FAAPMR, Jimmy D Bowen
MD, FAAPMR, CSCS, in The Sports Medicine
Resource Manual, 2008

Isometric contraction

Isometric contraction occurs when muscle length remains relatively constant as tension is produced. For example, during a biceps curl, holding the dumbbell in a constant/static position rather than actively raising or lowering it is an example of isometric contraction. Although the forces generated during isometric contractions are potentially greater than during concentric contractions, muscles are seldom injured during this type of contraction. Isometric exercises are often used during the early phases of rehabilitating a musculotendinous injury because the intensity of contraction and the muscle length at which it contracts can be controlled. Breathing increases blood and oxygen supply to your muscles, which in turn helps with

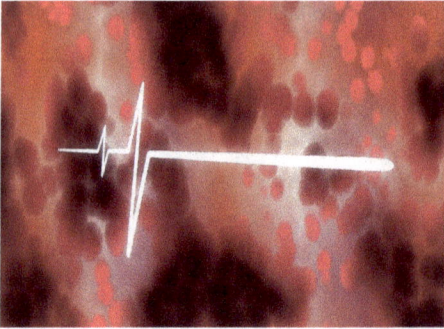

growth and endurance. In fact, famous martial artist Bruce Lee used these same techniques to prepare his body for the big screen.

Isometric Exercise Training

IET involves a single sustained muscle contraction against an immovable load or resistance with no, or minimal, change in length of the muscle group involved. An increasing body of evidence suggests that IET

70

promotes **significant reductions in resting systolic and DBPs** in hypertensive and normotensive men and women. Isometric hand grip training (IHG) has been shown to **improve resting blood flow** better than those observed in dynamic resistance training, dynamic aerobic exercise training, and training consisting of both dynamic resistance and aerobic activity.

BREATHING CORRECTLY

Breathing increases blood and oxygen supply to your muscles, which in turn helps with growth and endurance. In fact, famous martial artist Bruce Lee used these same techniques to prepare his body for the big screen.

1) Sipping Breath exercise

To start, stand in a fighter's pose.

Exhale air out of your lungs until they feel empty.

Then, tense up your whole body with a static contraction, or in other words, flexing in place.

At this point start your sipping breath, which consists of short, quick inhaled breaths. When you exhale, relax your muscles.

What's unique about isometric training is that your muscles are engaged for an extended period of your time throughout the movement, which makes it necessary for your muscles to recruit more muscle fibers. Consider holding a leg extension for 45 seconds compared to "repping- out" with 12-repetitions. Breathing becomes a particularly important part of the exercise. Holding your breath is NOT an option and should NEVER be done!

There is an enormous difference between your quadriceps being contracted for 45-seconds straight, instead of 2 seconds per rep, with a second 1 second of relaxation after you get to the tip of the movement. The longer the muscle is contracted, the more muscle fibers it will recruit. The more muscle fibers recruited, the higher the expansion of the whole muscle. Isometrics is an optimal workout for anyone from age 15-90. Anyone can use these exact isometric training techniques to spice up strength and stamina no matter your current age and physical shape. Isometrics don't seem to be only effective for building muscle mass and strength but they're also the safest form of exercise you'll be able to do because they put less stress on your joints than traditional exercises do.

One of the numerous benefits of exercise is that you just work both slow and fast twitch muscle fibers at the identical time, which are answerable for both strength and endurance...

A recent study shows the difference within the level of muscle activation during isometric, concentric, and eccentric muscle actions. Isometric exercises recruited 95.2% more muscle fibers. The eccentric movement of an exercise (lowering) recruited 88.3% and the concentric (lifting) movement recruited 89.7% muscle fibers. This gives isometrics a 5% advantage in fiber recruitment. Whether you're training for your next powerlifting competition or trying to beat arthritis, isometrics training has something for you.

Another recent study comparing the extent of muscle activation during isometric, concentric, and eccentric muscle actions found that an individual can recruit over 5% more motor-units/muscle fibers during a maximal isometric muscle movement during either a maximal eccentric (lowering) or maximal concentric (lifting) action; that's 95.2% for isometric compared to 88.3% for the eccentric and 89.7% for the concentric. These findings are in accordance with the body of literature that finds that someone can recruit most motor-units during a maximal isometric action. What this means is that isometric training can improve our ability to recruit motor units during a maximal contraction. within the future, this improved neural drive could greatly increase one's strength production potential! In the past, isometric exercises are described as a way that ought to only be used by advanced lifters.

One of the most important shortcomings of lower-class lifters is the incapacity to provide maximum intramuscular tension during a concentric contraction. Isometric exercise can thus be wont to find out how to supply this high level of tension, because it requires fewer motor skills than the corresponding dynamic action.

A STIMULUS FOR MUSCLE GROWTH

While initial reports on isometric action training hypothesized that this sort of coaching wouldn't cause significant muscle gains thanks to the absence of labor, recent findings indeed conclude that an isometric training regimen can cause gains in muscle size!

A study in (2002) found a mean muscle area (size) improvement of 12.4% for maximal isometric contraction training and of 5.3% for isometric training at 60% of maximum contraction after a training period of ten weeks.

The authors attributed the gain in muscle size to metabolic demands and endocrine activities instead of mechanical stress and neuromuscular control. It's important to notice that isometric exercises still have limitations. Yes, it can help increase strength and size, but without a concurrent dynamic (yielding and overcoming) program, the gains are slow. In fact, some coaches note that gains from isometric exercises stop after six to eight weeks of use. So, while isometric training will be extremely helpful to figure on

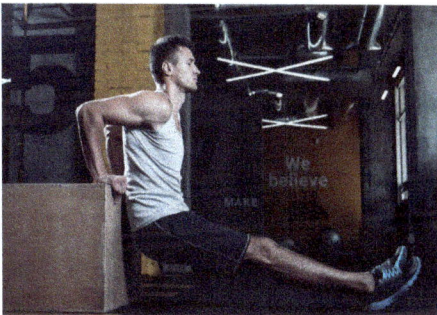

a liability or improve an athlete's capacity to activate motor-units, it should only be used for brief periods of your time when progress has over-involved or when a rapid strength

improvement is needed. Isometric training can even be useful in periods of lowered training volumes. Once you must decrease your training load either thanks to fatigue symptoms or time constraints, isometric work can help prevent muscle and strength losses.

THE "NEW" ISOMETRIC TRAINING

Many studies don't report lots of muscle growth from isometric training. This can be only because the old German model (Hettingter and Müller) of six-second actions was used in the first experiments. This duration of effort, albeit adequate for strength gains, isn't sufficient to cause hypertrophic changes within the muscles. In other words, it won't cause you to be big. This form of coaching is named maximal intensity isometric training and it's similar in effect to the maximal effort method (1-5 reps with 90-100% of your max), which ends up in strength gains with little, if any, muscle size gains.

However, using sets lasting 20 to 60 seconds will represent a crucial hypertrophy stimulus, similar in nature to the repetitive effort method (8-12 reps with 70-80% of your maximum). *Another key point is that the majority of studies performed on isometric training were short term, often using an insufficient period to stimulate a significant increase in muscle mass but sufficient to cause neural adaptations resulting in strength gains.*

In my findings Isometrics is NOT the best choice for building bigger muscles. The KEY to Isometrics is building Strength. With an increase in strength, you increase your weight thus you lift heavier and muscle size can and will occur. However, you will never achieve Arnold status with Isometrics. It's not for that. The fact is that steroids are eaten like candy to achieve that bloated bodybuilder physique.

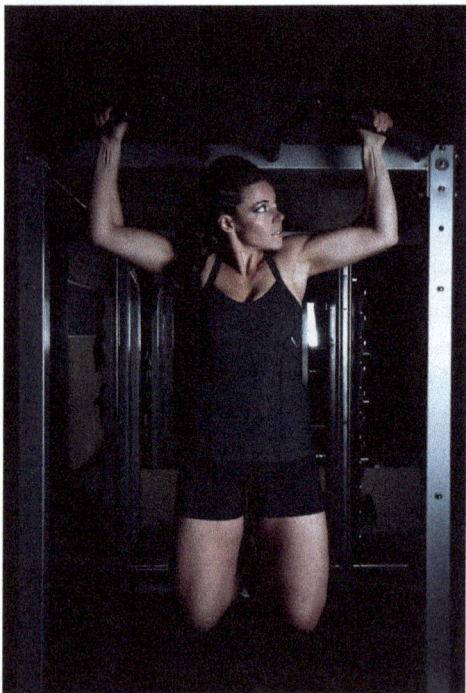

The programs in this book called **HYSOMETRICS**, I developed by using a combination of Isometrics and dynamic exercises with weights, Iso-Bow or Bands.

The concept for Hysometrics is to utilize the BEST of both worlds. The Strength training of ISOMETRICS with the Muscle building and toning of Weights/Reps.

I am confident that it will work for you. This is no sales pitch! This was developed by me after massive surgeries and radiation on my brain all in less than a year!

The Two designed programs in this book are:

HYSOMETRICS- Using a combination of ISOMETRICS, Weights/Bands/Iso-Bow in a single workout.

'RAPID REPS'- My Customized POWER LIFTING workout using anything other than Heavy Olympic weights in a gym.

Both Programs are way outside the box for this type of training. Sure, you could just lift weights, go through the motions. Most people do. After a while they just stop working out because they get hurt, see no growth or find themselves in the gym for 2 hours at a time. That won't happen with **HYSOMETRICS** or **'RAPID REPS'.**

NUTRITION/EATING RIGHT

You have heard it all before, EATING PROPERLY is the right way to get your mind and body into shape. I'm here to tell you that without a doubt, there is no more factual statement in the world! To be honest, if you have no plans to alter your diet, then you can stop reading right now.

NOTHING you do will work!

Without eating the proper foods, you are just adding calories to your body that it cannot burn up! Think of it as FUEL! Food is basically FUEL to keep your body active.

The human body can only TAKE IN so many calories per day!

The **FIRST** thing you need to do is go to the many Calorie Count calculators online and type in your Height, Age, Weight and Activity Level. It will calculate how many calories your body needs to keep weight and to lose weight. Do you need to count the calories going in? That depends on if you are serious about losing weight. I memorized the FOOD CHARTS. I could tell you exactly how many calories my breakfast was, my Dinner and any snack I had.

A good calculator should look something like this!

I LOST 70 Pounds. Even today I can keep my weight within **3 pounds** of my target on any given day! Your **CALORIE INTAKE NUMBER** is the most Important number you will have in the battle to lose or maintain your weight!

The Fact that food today have so much CRAP in them is a REAL problem. HIGH-FRUCTOSE CORN SYRUP in my opinion is the BIGGEST POISON you can put in your mouth. And it's in EVERYTHING! No wonder diabetes is out of control.

The World Health Organization (WHO) estimates that 90 percent of people around the world who have diabetes have type 2.

While that sounds a little high to me, it shows that we certainly have a problem and **HIGH-FRUCTOSE CORN SYRUP is right in the middle of that!**

So, Nutrition is Important?

No, I didn't say that! NUTRITION is the **MOST IMPORTANT!**

Unless you want to start powerlifting eating three cheeseburgers at a sitting and deadlift 600 lbs. I don't see that working!

I'll give you an example. The World's Strongest man eats, and this is NO LIE!

10,000 calories (about 800 minutes of running) a day!! The average person maxes out 2,000 calories a day!

They make Dieting out to be so COMPLEX... It's NOT!

In fact, dieting is VERY SIMPLE!! One rule that I will tell you to follow!

TAKE IN LESS CALORIES
THAN YOUR BODY NEEDS!
That's IT!
That is the million-dollar piece of advice that NO ONE TELLS YOU!

It's not about buying premade foods, joining food clubs that's all-MARKETING BULLSHIT!

Get your daily calorie number and take in LESS calories than you should. RESULT:

WEIGHT LOSS!

Remember you are always burning calories. Doing housework, driving, even reading at your desk. Your body is still burning calories. Know your body! Use food as FUEL! Do your basic workouts!

Take in just what you NEED! And you'll be shocked at how fast you will drop the weight

FYI. In my Power Lifting days, I would consume **5,000-6,000** calories a day at a body weight of 245 lbs. At 24 years old, I burned that off with no problem. In fact, I could eat up to **7,000 calories** a day and still not put on weight.

That was THEN…..This is NOW :)
In fact, after my back surgery, I was still eating around 4,000 calories a day. I had no one to blame for ballooning to 280 pounds!

Much of this program involves **THINKING!**

- **Thinking about HOW you will approach this.**
- **Thinking about HOW you will execute.**
- **Thinking about HOW you will change your schedule**
- **Thinking about HOW you will change your lifestyle.**

When I say HYSOMETRICS is for the body and mind, I TRULY mean you have to use BOTH to reach your goals! This program is as much for your mind as it is your body. I want to see people take an Intelligent, Cerebral approach to fixing their body and mind! Make no mistake, if your head is NOT INTO the program, this will NEVER WORK. Going through the motions has NEVER gotten people into shape and it NEVER will! You have to dedicate yourself to the cause. Set a goal and go for it!

Nutrition means eating a quart of Peanut Butter Cup Ice Cream is NOT an option. If you do, and it happens, just count those calories against your daily number! You may have to ride the bike an extra 20 minutes, but you can do that!

I LOVED Ice Cream, Whoopie Pies, Hershey Chocolate!! I haven't had any of that for almost 3 years now! I don't miss the sugar at all!

As a guy that ate 6,000 calories a day, I ate EVERYTHING! For me to tell you what to eat would be hypocritical and I hate hypocrites!

With that said you must start here. DECIDE that you want to lose 5,10, 20 pounds, and stick to it!

There is NO WAY IN HELL losing weight is EASY.

Exactly why anyone that talks about losing weight or a new fad diet becomes a gazillionaire in the first year. Problem is,

NONE OF THOSE FAD DIETS WORK! WHAT DOES WORK ?

Using your Mind to convince your body that. **YOU CAN DO THIS!**

Throwing on a pair of old sweats and working out like you were 22 again! Losing weight and toning up your body is like a part time job. If you are over 50 it's a **FULL TIME JOB!**

NO, not everyone can do it!

I know that you are not just ANYONE! You purchased this book for a reason. You don't want to be like all the others.

TO ME, that means you have what it takes to follow through!

- **THINK**
- **PLAN**
- **EXECUTE**
- **RETHINK**
- **ADAPT**
- **EVALUATE**

Now, what are you waiting for?

Tip Library

Use the *Start Simple with MyPlate* tips below or create your own tips that support the MyPlate food group messages. Share these tips on your social media channels or incorporate them into your promotional activities.

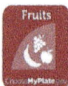

FOCUS ON WHOLE FRUITS

1. Include fruit at breakfast! Top whole-grain cereal with your favorite fruit, add berries to pancakes, or mix dried fruit into hot oatmeal.

2. Try a new fruit for a snack. Fruits vary in vitamins and minerals so mix it up!

3. Add your favorite fresh or canned fruit to a salad or enjoy as a side.

4. Keep a bowl of whole fruit on the table, counter, or in the refrigerator.

5. On long car trips, pack fruit to snack on! Bananas, apples, grapes, and plums all travel well, as do dried fruit such as raisins, cranberries or apricots.

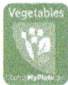

VARY YOUR VEGGIES

1. Cook a variety of colorful veggies. Make extra vegetables and save some for later. Use them for a stew, soup, or a pasta dish.

2. Make each meal colorful by adding red, dark-green, yellow, or orange vegetables to your plate.

92

3. Use dark leafy greens, like romaine lettuce and spinach, to make salads. Add red and orange veggies for extra color and nutrition!

4. Cook it once, eat twice. Make extra vegetables and save some for later.

5. Vary your veggies by adding a new vegetable to a different meal each day.

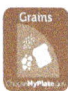

MAKE HALF YOUR GRAINS WHOLE GRAINS

1. Add brown rice to your stir-fry dishes. Combine your favorite veggies and protein foods for a nutritious meal!

2. Use whole-grain bread when making a sandwich. If you choose refined-grain bread, make sure it's enriched by checking the ingredients list.

3. Pack a whole-grain snack for work or when you're on the go. Whole-grain cereal or crackers and plain popcorn are great choices!

4. Mix whole-grain cereal with nuts and dried fruit for a great afternoon snack.

5. Try something new—choose less common whole grains (amaranth, quinoa, millet, and triticale). Look for recipes online.

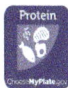

VARY YOUR PROTEIN ROUTINE

1. Next taco night, try adding a new protein, like shrimp, beans, or beef.

2. Make colorful kabobs with your favorite protein foods and veggies! Enjoy the kabobs grilled or roasted.

3. Serve seafood twice a week—it's simple! Make patties with canned salmon, crab, or tuna, or use them on a seafood sandwich.

4. Enjoy hard-cooked eggs as a snack, on salads, or in main dishes.

5. Make beans, peas, and soy products part of your meals often. Try black bean burgers, hummus, or stir-fried tofu.

MOVE TO LOW-FAT OR FAT-FREE MILK OR YOGURT

93

Dairy

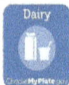

1. Enjoy a low-fat yogurt parfait for breakfast. Top with fruit and nuts to get in two more food groups.

2. Be a role model! Parents and caregivers who drink milk and eat dairy foods show kids that it is important for their health.

3. Leave room for some milk in your morning caffeine routine. Make or order your coffee, latte, or cappuccino with low-fat milk.

4. Cook your oatmeal or other hot cereal in fat-free or low-fat milk instead of water.

5. To get calcium at lunch, add cheese to your sandwich. When choosing dairy products, fat-free and low-fat dairy are good options.

Limit

DRINK AND EAT BEVERAGES AND FOOD WITH LESS SODIUM, SATURATED FAT, AND ADDED SUGARS

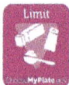

Salt and Sodium

1. Taste your food before you reach for the salt shaker. Spices and herbs are a great way to add extra flavor.

2. Cook at home! Preparing your own food helps you decide the amount of salt used in meals.

Saturated Fat

1. Trim visible fat from meat before cooking or remove the skin from poultry to reduce saturated fat.

2. Try a bean chili or roll up a tortilla with hummus and veggies for a low-saturated fat meal.

Added Sugars

1. Help kids learn about added sugars in foods. Read the ingredients and compare different foods together.

2. Fruits can help you satisfy your sweet cravings. Make it fun with a fruit kabob using bananas, apples, pears, and orange sections.

94

10 tips

*Nutrition
Education Series*

healthy eating for an active lifestyle

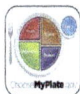

10 tips for combining good nutrition and physical activity

For youth and adults engaging in physical activity and sports, healthy eating is essential for optimizing performance. Combining good nutrition with physical activity can lead to a healthier lifestyle.

1 maximize with nutrient-packed foods
Give your body the nutrients it needs by eating a variety of nutrient-packed food, including whole grains, lean protein, fruits and vegetables, and low-fat or fat-free dairy. Eat less food high in solid fats, added sugars, and sodium (salt).

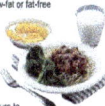

2 energize with grains
Your body's quickest energy source comes from foods such as bread, pasta, oatmeal, cereals, and tortillas. Be sure to make at least half of your grain food choices whole-grain foods like whole-wheat bread or pasta and brown rice.

3 power up with protein
Protein is essential for building and repairing muscle. Choose lean or low-fat cuts of beef or pork, and skinless chicken or turkey. Get your protein from seafood twice a week. Quality protein sources come from plant-based foods, too.

4 mix it up with plant protein foods
Variety is great! Choose beans and peas (kidney, pinto, black, or white beans; split peas; chickpeas; hummus), soy products (tofu, tempeh, veggie burgers), and unsalted nuts and seeds.

5 vary your fruits and vegetables
Get the nutrients your body needs by eating a variety of colors, in various ways. Try blue, red, or black berries; red and yellow peppers; and dark greens like spinach and kale. Choose fresh, frozen, low-sodium canned, dried, or 100 percent juice options.

6 don't forget dairy
Foods like fat-free and low-fat milk, cheese, yogurt, and fortified soy beverages (soymilk) help to build and maintain strong bones needed for everyday activities.

7 balance your meals
Use MyPlate as a reminder to include all food groups each day. Learn more at www.ChooseMyPlate.gov.

8 drink water
Stay hydrated by drinking water instead of sugary drinks. Keep a reusable water bottle with you to always have water on hand.

9 know how much to eat
Get personalized nutrition information based on your age, gender, height, weight, current physical activity level, and other factors. Use SuperTracker to determine your calorie needs, plan a diet that's right for you, and track progress toward your goals. Learn more at www.SuperTracker.usda.gov.

10 reach your goals
Earn Presidential recognition for reaching your healthy eating and physical activity goals. Log on to www.presidentschallenge.org to sign up for the Presidential Active Lifestyle Award (PALA+).

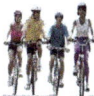

Go to www.ChooseMyPlate.gov and www.Fitness.gov for more information.

DG TipSheet No. 25
March 2013
Center for Nutrition Policy and Promotion
USDA is an equal opportunity provider and employer.

My Physical Activity Diary

Monday		
Time of Day	Description of Activity (Type and Intensity Level)	Duration

Tuesday		
Time of Day	Description of Activity (Type and Intensity Level)	Duration

Wednesday		
Time of Day	Description of Activity (Type and Intensity Level)	Duration

Thursday		
Time of Day	Description of Activity (Type and Intensity Level)	Duration

Friday		
Time of Day	Description of Activity (Type and Intensity Level)	Duration

Saturday		
Time of Day	Description of Activity (Type and Intensity Level)	Duration

Sunday		
Time of Day	Description of Activity (Type and Intensity Level)	Duration

Notes:

Learn more at https://www.cdc.gov/healthyweight/losing_weight/eating_habits.html

CDC

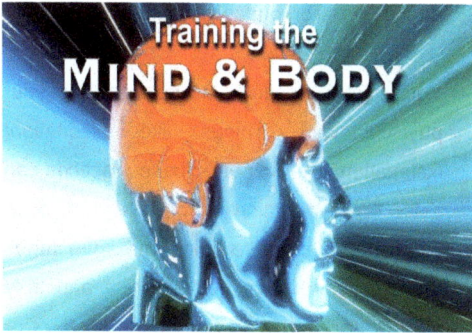

Training the
MIND & BODY

Connecting the Mind and Body

The connection between your physical and mental health.. It includes factors like your emotions, social interactions, belief system, and behavior. Each of those influences your well-being.. Let's say that you're having a rotten day at work where nothing seems to travel your way. Many times we have a Bad day. Consider how your mood will affect the remainder of your day and your performance during your workout as a result.

Your mental health is as important as your physical self. Things like Meditation, Relaxation, Therapy etc. These practices can settle down your mind in order that you'll focus better on what you're doing. the advantages go far beyond work and exercise and truly have large impacts on your health.

Exercise stimulates the Mind-Body Connection. The nerve cells or **neurons** in your brain communicate with one another using chemicals called neurotransmitters. And even more brilliant is the proven fact that intense exercise can increase levels of two important chemicals. To explore this concept, participants found out at 85 percent of their maximum pulse rate for 20 minutes. The researchers used MRI imaging to test levels of glutamate and gamma-aminobutyric acid

(GABA) before and after workouts. They found significant increases once they were tested within three minutes after understanding compared to the group that didn't. That means better communication between nerve cells and a possible therapy for treating depression. That's not the sole brain health good thing about regular workouts. Exercise can help maintain good brain health while you age and should even improve your memory.

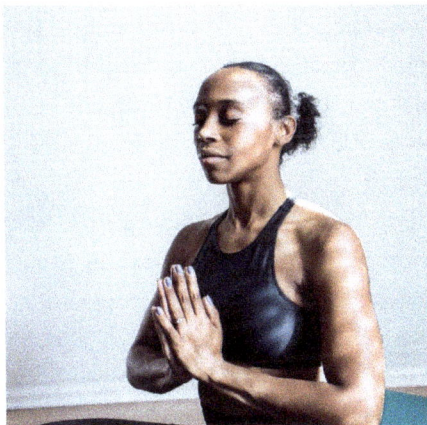

'ISO 7 DAY INTRO' PROGRAM:

We can talk all day and night about Isometrics and how effective a workout is. Until you actually do the exercises you cannot judge how your body will react. Unlike Dynamic lifting exercises, Isometrics incorporates many more body functions. Along with muscle tension, Isometrics utilizes the tendons, ligaments and nervous system all at the same time. It takes time for the body to get used to accessing not only the muscle but the nerves as well. Exactly why I developed the 7 DAY Intro Program. In just a brief time you can get your body used to ISOMETRICS and how it will work for you.

During the first 7 Days, We are going to teach the brain and the body the new way to train. Unlike weight Lifting, Isometrics does not break down the muscle in such a violent manner. Actually there are those people that believe you can do ISOMETRICS on a daily basis. Knowing how muscle works and the time a muscle needs to recuperate. I don't suggest that. I like to teach others that a solid 24-48 hours between workouts is best. For those over fifty years of age, working out 3 times a week is a must. By fifty you have lost a good amount of muscle mass. To compensate, working out three times a week is very helpful.

So, What is this '7 DAY INTRO' Basically, it's getting your body and mind used to the ISOMETRIC process. For the first seven days I want you to practice Isometrics EVERYDAY. Yea, I know I just said that rest is needed. You will rest after the initial 7 days.

I suggest you pick 2 exercises for each body part: You can refer to the chart. We are ONLY doing ISOMETRICS. **ISOMETRIC EXERCISE ONLY! Always start with large body parts first. The right sequence would be:**

LEGS

BACK

CHEST

SHOULDERS

TRICEPS

BICEPS

ABS

INTRO PROCEDURE:

- Pick the same time each day
- Pick 2 exercises per body part.
- Only do 2 sets of 10 second holds
- Tension is between 70-100% of full strength
- :30 second rest between
- NO SUPERSETS (set then rest,)
- Alternate Exercises each day
- Keep a journal for the 7 days
- **TOTAL BODY** workout **(ALL BODY PARTS)**

The emphasis is on doing the proper form, timing, and breathing for each exercise.

Your first couple of days should NOT be at FULL 100% exertion. Start out with around 60-70% of your full strength. HOLD BACK just a bit!!

Day 3 you can slowly increase your intensity. Should you ever get confused there are examples on my blog. Feel free to contact me if you still need help.
What should you expect?

After 7 days you will most likely be a bit sore, nothing like lifting weights. You'll have an idea on how Isometrics works. You will also warm up your ligaments, muscles and tendons for a HYSOMETRIC workout. This is VERY IMPORTANT. Tearing a tendon, muscle or ligament has a long recovery time. We NEVER want to see that happen. Write down exactly what you did for each exercise.

Day 1-7. You will go back to this log to see what was effective, what hurt (if anything) and what work for your body. After the 7-day Intro, I feel that you can begin the HYSOMETRIC Hybrid workout.

HYSOMETRIC BEGINNERS PROGRAM:

The 'Hysometric' program is designed for individuals that are new to Isometric training. This beginning program is suited for people with prior Injuries and or disabilities. The goal is to build strength, NOT BIG MUSCLES.

The Basic Hysometric Program will take around 20 minutes to complete. This is a Total Body Program. Meaning all body parts are trained in one day, at one time. For those over 50 years old it is recommended that you work out 3 times a week doing this program. Because of the muscle response in people over 50, training the muscle 3 times a week helps reverse any muscle loss you may have.

The HYSOMETRIC PROGRAM doesn't care if you are young or old, black, white, or green, fat or skinny. All you need is the will to want to get into better shape.

'RAPID REPS' POWER PROGRAM:

The 'Rapid Reps' program is designed for individuals that have done some weight training, have seen no growth, no increase in size or strength. The overall concept of 'Rapid Reps' is to mimic the POWERLIFTING workout using a form of Isometrics called

'OVERCOMING ISOMETRICS'. Which is basically you trying to move or lift an IMMOVABLE OBJECT quickly! I developed the idea as an ex competitive powerlifter that didn't have access to Olympic plates. I found the workout to be just as intense as maxing a single heavy rep.

ISOMETRIC REP BREATHING

When doing isometrics exercises, you will struggle to take deep breaths in and out, and you should not, NEVER, NEVER HOLD YOUR BREATH!
If you try and breathe too deeply you will end up slipping out of the movement and probably collapsing on the floor.

Keeping your breathing shallow will enable you to keep your trunk tight because you are full of air, you are always pulling oxygen into your blood, and you can then hold for a lot longer.

Air cycles around your nose and mouth but it will create movement around your lungs too. You will continuously move air in and out of your lungs without a lot of effort because you can keep your muscles tight.

How to:

- Start with a nice big breath as you get into the hold, starting with full lungs will help keep them full.

- As your whole body tightens, start to take shallow breaths through your nose and mouth.

- When your body starts trembling you will notice your breath cycling to that rhythm

- Bringing the air into your nose and mouth, combined with your body movement allows for very little diaphragm movement, instead you are cycling air in and around your lungs continuously.

HOW TO PERFORM ISOMETRIC POWER BREATHING EXERCISE

I. Before arising from your bed, lie on your back and relax together with your hands at your sides.

2. Inhale deeply through your nostrils and imagine that you are filling your entire body right down to your toes with enriched oxygen. Literally, let yourself expand.

3. Once you can inhale no farther, hold for a count of 7 seconds, while pulling in your abdominal muscles, then begin to exhale.

4. During the exhale, squeeze your abdominal muscles as
though you are wringing water from a wet towel. Squeeze the entire rectus abdominis from top to bottom as tightly as possible, while making an IISSSSS " or "fffff" sound.

5. When you have achieved peak intensity or contraction of the abdominals, hold for 7 or more seconds, squeezing until your exhale is completely finished. leave nothing in your lungs. Try to get everything out.

6. While performing step 5, it is a healthy practice to contract or pull your perineum up and inward. This will not only improve your overall energy, but greatly improve sexual function as well.

7. Perform this Isometric Power Breathing exercise 10 times in succession before getting

out of bed. You are then welcome to get up, stand before an open window, and do more of the same. You can also do this exercise anytime throughout the day to release mental stress and to recharge and energize.

THE RIGHT WAY TO BREATHE DURING EXERCISE

The gold standard during strength training is to inhale on relaxation and exhale during exertion. For cardio, you generally breathe in and out through the nose or, when intensity ramps up, through the mouth.

✓ DO NOT hold your breath, count each rep aloud, to avoid holding your breath

✓ Try exhaling during the left foot fall (not the right).

✓ If you can't catch his breath, stand tall with your hands behind your head to open the lungs and allow for deeper inhalations—don't bend over with hands on knees.

✓ When cooling down or stretching, deep, slow breathing helps calm the body and aid in recovery.

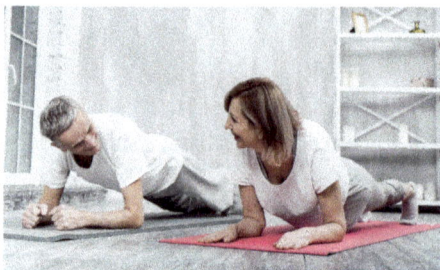

Since this is a book about how to give yourself strength, and the kind of body you have always dreamed of having, you must visualize in your mind the type of physique you want to have. Do you want to dramatically enhance the size of your muscles? Or do you want to achieve a lean, ripped look? Define your goals from day one, even before you start working out!. The first part of the workout is training your mind to believe in what you are doing. Tell yourself "You can do this" "You will reach your goals" and Most Importantly ALWAYS remind yourself by saying to yourself EVERYDAY.

"I can do ANTHING I set my mind to; I can achieve anything I desire."

Repeat this to yourself Every day.

When waking up, in the shower, while driving. Train your mind to believe in YOU! Whatever your choice, it can be achieved with the methods outlined in this book.

The only way you can achieve success is to keep reminding yourself that you are able to achieve success!

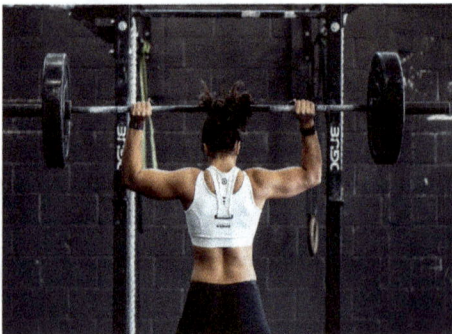

3 Keys to all of these Exercises

I. Programming the right thoughts into your mind. POSITIVE REMINDERS

2. Focus on them. Constantly Repeat your goals to yourself.

3. See yourself reaching your goals, ALWAYS follow through. We NEVER QUIT!

Before we start, I want to share with you what I believe to be the most important piece of equipment to perform ISOMETRICS I have ever seen. The ISO-BOW is the ultimate Isometric tool. Portable, Inexpensive and Effective. I recommend that you order this gem to perform some of the workouts I have outlined in this book!

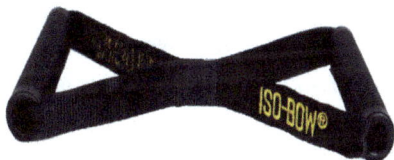

The **MOST IMPORTANT** piece of Isometric equipment you can own.

The **Bull Worker ISO-BOW** is the $20 dollar piece of gear that will pay for itself 1,000 times over! I continue to use mine 3 times a week!

When I first saw this little wonder, I knew Immediately that I would be able to do all of the Basic Isometric Exercises and be able to make up new ones. I can throw this in my bag and do a complete workout no matter where I am! I have even done a complete arm workout while riding in the cab on the way to the airport. In a word the Iso-Bow is 'AMAZING'

Big Thank You to Bull Worker John and Chrisman Hughes for allowing me to post this chart. If there is only 1 piece of equipment that you can buy, **BUY THIS FIRST!**

https://www.bullworker.com/iso-bow/

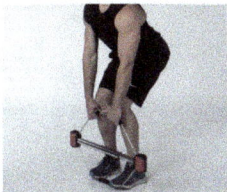

DEADLIFT

Muscles Engaged: Lower Back -
Quadriceps - Glutes - Hamstrings
• Place both feet securely on bottom
  cable. Bend knees. Keep your
  back straight. Spread cables in a
  squatting manner.
*Do not exceed maximum compression

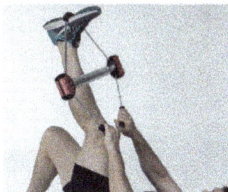

ONE LEG PRESS
(BOTH SIDES)

Muscles Engaged: Quadriceps -
Glutes - Hamstrings
• Place foot securely in cable.
• Keep arms still. Press with your leg.
*Do not exceed maximum compression

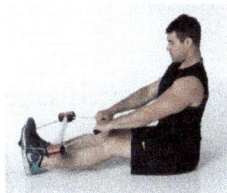

DEADLIFT (GROUND)

Muscles Engaged: Lower Back -
Quadriceps - Glutes - Hamstrings
• Place both feet securely on bottom
  cable. Bend knees slightly. Keep
  your back straight. Rise using lower
  back.

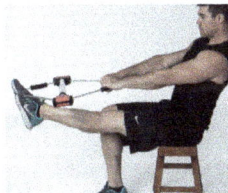

CALF EXTENSION
(BOTH SIDES)

Muscles Engaged: Calves
• Place foot securely through cable.
• Point toes.
*Ensure toe is always pointed to keep
cable secure.

117

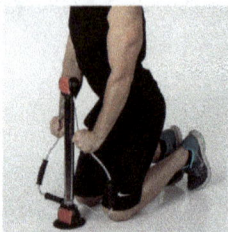

TRICEPS CABLE PUSH DOWN

Muscles Engaged: Triceps
- Keep your back straight. Push bottom cables down.
- Bend only at your elbows.
- Secure Bullworker placement using your non-slip pad.

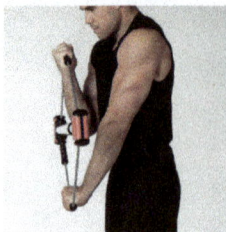

TRICEPS PUSH DOWN (BOTH SIDES)

Muscles Engaged: Triceps
- Ensure hand grips are placed in the middle of the cables
- Bend only at your elbow. Push bottom cable down.

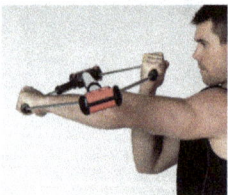

TRICEPS EXTENSION (BOTH SIDES)

Muscles Engaged: Triceps
- Ensure hand grips are placed in the middle of the cables.
- Bend only at your elbow. Extend cable out.

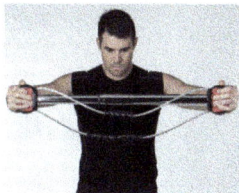

CHEST COMPRESSION

Muscles Engaged: Chest -
Shoulders
• Ensure elbows are parallel to
  the ground.
• Compress your Bow Classic.

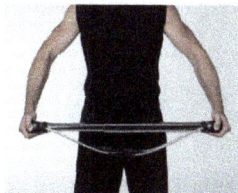

CHEST COMPRESSION
(LOWER)

Muscles Engaged: Chest -
Shoulders
• Compress your Bow Classic at
  or below your waist.

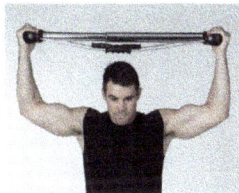

CHEST COMPRESSION
(UPPER)

Muscles Engaged: Chest -
Shoulders
• Compress your Bow Classic at
  or above shoulder height.

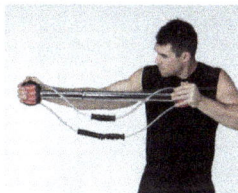

SIDE CHEST COMPRESSION
(BOTH SIDES)

Muscles Engaged: Chest - Shoulders
- Triceps
• Extend one arm fully. Compress
  your Bow Classic with your opposite
  arm.

119

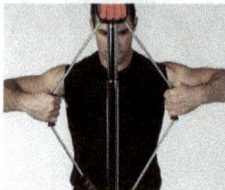

CABLE SPREAD

Muscles Engaged: Upper Back -
Posterior Deltoids
• Ensure hand grips are placed in the
  middle of the cables.
• Keep your elbows parallel to the
  ground. Spread both cables evenly.

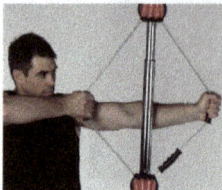

ARCHER (BOTH SIDES)

Muscles Engaged: Upper Back
• Ensure hand grips are placed in the
  middle of the cables and elbows are
  parallel to the ground
• Extend one arm. Spread cable using
  opposite arm.

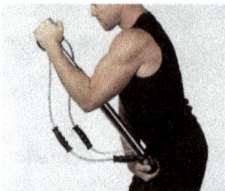

LAT PULL DOWN
(BOTH SIDES)

Muscles Engaged: Lats - Back
• Ensure hand grip is placed securely
  on your upper thigh.
• In a straight motion pull down.

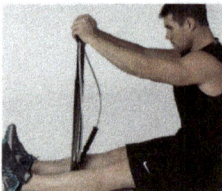

SEATED LAT PUSH DOWN

Muscles Engaged: Lats - Back
• Place Bow Classic securely
  on non-slip pad with arms
  extended

120

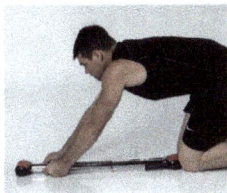

PLANK CRUNCH

Muscles Engaged: Abs - Lower Back
• Place the Bow Classic in front of your knees. Perform a crunch (keep arms straight).

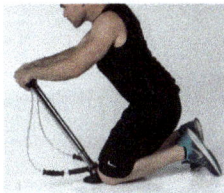

RESISTED CRUNCH

Muscles Engaged: Abs - Lower Back
• Place the Bow Classic on your non-slip pad in front. Perform a crunch (keep arms straight).
*Variation, stand and place on secure raised surface. Perform crunch.

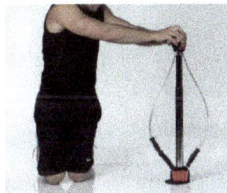

UPRIGHT RESISTED CRUNCH (BOTH SIDES)

Muscles Engaged: Abs - Lower Back
• Place the Bow Classic on your non-slip pad away from your body. Perform a crunch (keep arms straight).

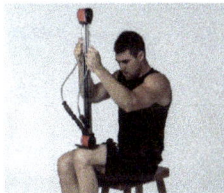

SEATED LOWER AB RAISE (BOTH SIDES)

Muscles Engaged: Lower Abs - Hip Flexor
• Place non-slip pad on knee.
• Hold cables securely. Raise your knee keeping your arms in place.

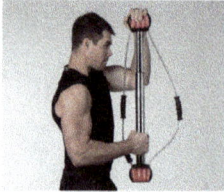

HAMMER BICEPS CURL (BOTH SIDES)

Muscles Engaged: Biceps
- Grip lower tube.
- Keep upper arm still. Curl upwards bending only at elbow.

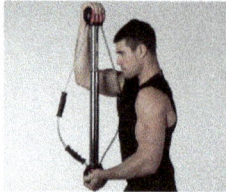

BICEPS CURL (BOTH SIDES)

Muscles Engaged: Biceps
- Place both hands on handles. Keep upper arm still. Curl upwards bending only at elbow.

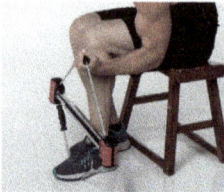

CONCENTRATION BICEPS CURL (BOTH SIDES)

Muscles Engaged: Biceps
- Place foot securely in cable.
- Curl bending only at the elbow.

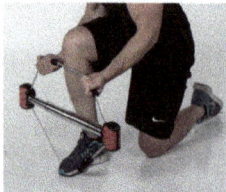

BICEPS CABLE CURL (KNEELING)

Muscles Engaged: Biceps
- Securely step on the bottom cable in a kneeling position
- Curl bending only at elbows.

Another cool little product is Activ5.
Portable, small and very smart!

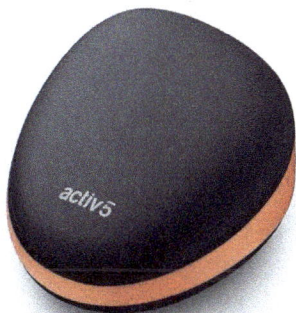

activ5.

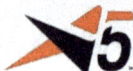

Activbody **Activ5 Challenge** Testimonial Study:

The Effect of the Activ5 Fitness Challenge on Total Body Appearance, Pant and Dress Size, Body Fat Mass and Weight Loss for Normal, Overweight, and Obese Men and Women. Eddie Gaut & Dr. Bob Girandola, ITG, a division of Detaug Testing Centers. Nov 19th 2016.

Electromyography Muscle Activity: A Single Activ5 Exercise vs. Treadmill Workout, Indoor Cycle, Squats, Lunges and Abdominal Crunches. Eddie Gaut, Detaug Testing Center. December 2016.

MUSCLE GAIN & FAT LOSS

+30%
STRENGTH INCREASE OVER 6 WEEKS

• On average, Activ5 Challenge participants increased their strength by 30% over 6 weeks.

That's the equivalent of 5% increase in strength per week.

62-71%
OF THE WEIGHT LOSS
IS PURE BODY FAT

• On average, 71% of the weight lost from top performing Activ5 Challenge participants was pure body fat.

• On average, 62% of the weight lost from all Activ5 Challenge participants was pure body fat.

124

activ5

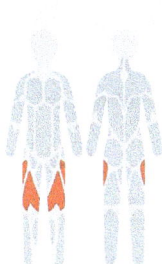

MUSCLE ACTIVITY VS GYM EXERCISES

• On average, Activ5 Challenge participants generated 39% more Quad muscle activity than squats, 37% more than lunges, 59% more than a treadmill workout and 59% more than indoor cycling.

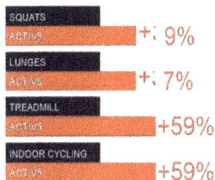

SQUATS / ACTIV5	+39%
LUNGES / ACTIV5	+37%
TREADMILL / ACTIV5	+59%
INDOOR CYCLING / ACTIV5	+59%

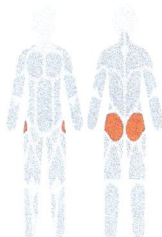

• On average, Activ5 Challenge participants generated 25% more Buttocks muscle activity than squats, 33% more than lunges, 42% more than a treadmill workout and 50% more than indoor cycling.

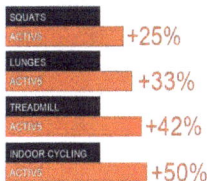

SQUATS / ACTIV5	+25%
LUNGES / ACTIV5	+33%
TREADMILL / ACTIV5	+42%
INDOOR CYCLING / ACTIV5	+50%

The Activ5 just may be the coolest little Isometric machine that you will ever use!

FYI

In your 30s, you start to lose muscle mass and function. The cause is age-related sarcopenia or sarcopenia with aging.

Physically inactive people can lose as much as 3% to 5% of their muscle mass each decade after age 30.

Even if you are active, you'll still have some muscle loss.

There's no test or specific level of muscle mass that will diagnose sarcopenia. Any loss of muscle matters because it lessens strength and mobility.

Sarcopenia typically happens faster around age 75. But it may also speed up as early as 65! It's a factor in frailty and the likelihood of falls and fractures in older adults.

SIMPLE HAND/FOREARM STRENGTH:

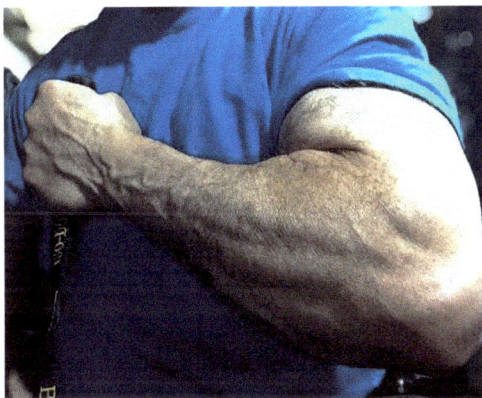

TARGETED MUSCLES:
GRIP/FOREARM/FINGERS

For many of us, as we are getting older the first thing, we find is our hands are just not as strong as when we were 25! Makes sense, we are losing muscle fiber and strength. Everything we do requires our hands and some sort of grip. The natural first move would be to make sure you strengthen your grip.

This one little exercise can be done while sitting in your favorite chair watching tv or on your drive to work, just twice a week takes about 5 minutes.

Using one simple tool EVERYONE has:

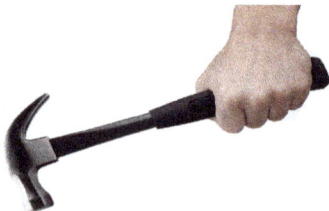

Go out to the toolbox and grab your hammer. Have a seat and take a couple deep breaths. You REALLY have to teach your brain to talk to the muscle. In this case the forearm, hand and fingers.

Grip Hammer with one hand, exhale and squeeze the hammer as tight as you can.

HOLD...HOLD...HOLD. Exhale every second of the two slowly. Hold the grip for 10 seconds, as hard as you can!
 BREATHE out as you count, with short breaths. Hold until 10...Switch hands.

Rest 1 minute after both hands have held for 10 seconds. Repeat.

You will want to do this 3 times for each hand.

Do this twice a week. After 3 weeks. you will notice a **minimum of 15% more strength in**

your hands and grip! You can add a third day and longer holds as you gain strength. Something so SIMPLE will make your life that much easier. That is WHY I LOVE ISOMETRICS!

FYI: *Don't have a hammer? Use a pipe, tennis ball, etc....I often do these on my steering wheel while driving.*
3 sets takes about 5 minutes!

THE WORKOUTS

Below, I have outlined some of the basic exercises that you can do with and without equipment. To begin I suggest choosing **TWO** exercises per **BODY PART** to 'superset' with. Keep in mind one of the important principles of **HYSOMETRICS** is to constantly change your workouts. Rotating the exercise is a great idea.

THE BASIC WORKOUT EXERCISES

LEGS:

The following Leg workout is for upper and lower leg muscles. This move is done in a 'SUPERSET FASHION' or two exercises done back-to-back with NO REST in between.

MOVEMENT:

Isometric wall squat
Sit up and put the bottom of your feet together. Place your hands on your ankles (not toes) 2. Take a deep breath in, exhale as you stretch forward with a straight back. Press your knees downward as you try to touch your knees to the floor, arms are slightly in front of your legs.

Quickly, sit on the floor with both toes touching the same wall. Push out with your toes until you are pushing your toes as if to be pushing the wall back. Hold that position for 10 seconds. Then relax.

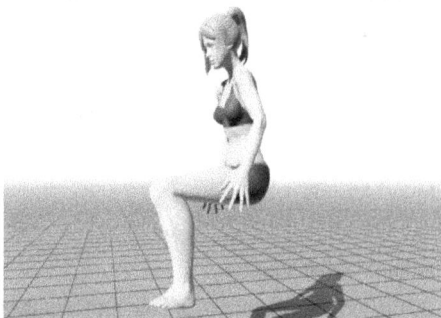

That is Set number one of three. Rest for 30 seconds then repeat Wall Squat and Calf Squeeze.

Leg Lift against hand pushing down

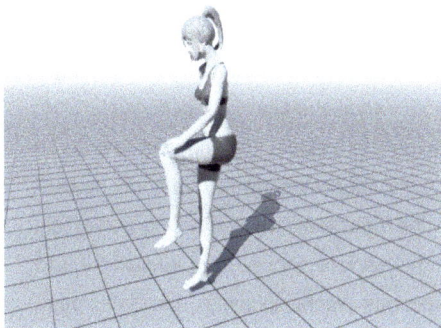

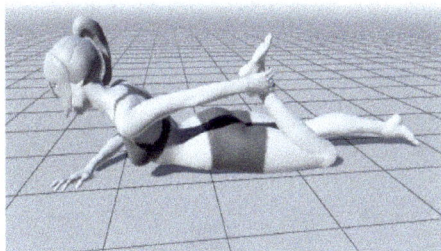

Quad Push- holding leg

Leg Curl using opposite leg.

Lie face down (as shown) with your feet close together and head raised, resting your weight on your hands and elbows. Place your left foot over your right ankle, keeping your feet about 3" off the floor (as shown). Pull firmly upward with the right foot, while resisting powerfully with the left foot. Slowly build tension for 3 to 4 seconds while inhaling. Maintain peak contraction for 7 to 12 seconds while slowly exhaling and making an f-f-f-f or 5-5-5-5 sound. Slowly release tension while breathing in and then completely relax while power breathing. Switch legs and repeat.

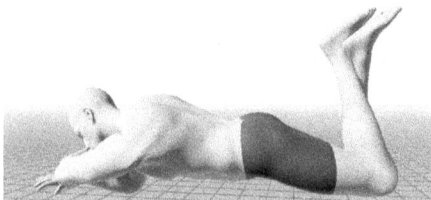

CALF RAISE

Keeping your heels on the floor. Flex your foot (as shown) and hold for about 10-15 seconds. You can also do this stretch by hanging your heels off the edge of a curb or step.

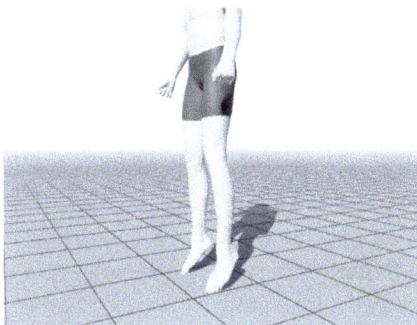

WALL CALF SQUEEZE

Find a wall and stand a few inches away. Put the toes of your right foot against the wall, keeping your heel on the floor. Flex your foot (as shown) and hold for about 10-15 seconds, then switch feet. You can also do this stretch by hanging your heels off the edge of a curb or step.

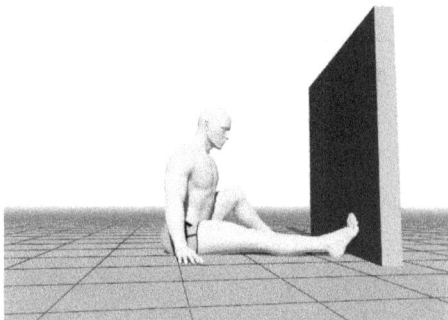

BACK- Option 1
WITHOUT EQUIPMENT MONKEY BAR, RAFTER, TREE BRANCH

Pull yourself up until your upper chest is level with the bar. Keep your chest puffed out, elbows pulled down and back, and focus on squeezing the shoulder blades together hard. Now hold it right there. The muscles burning in your upper back?

The Lower back row is a great exercise for developing the back muscles. ISO Row: Take a seat and bend your legs so you can reach and choke up on the towel. Pull the towel towards you and keep your shoulders down and away from your ears; this will allow you to not only feel your arms but also the lats and rear deltoids. Hold for 6-8 sec, relax for 2-3 seconds and repeat. You should be contracting about 80% of your max effort. Do 8 repetitions.

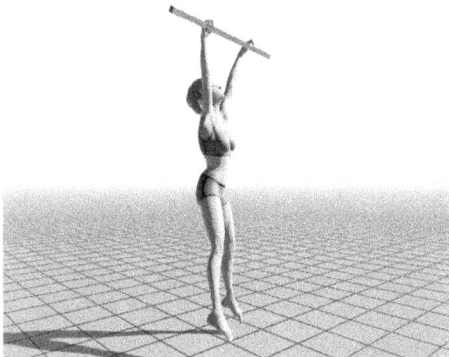

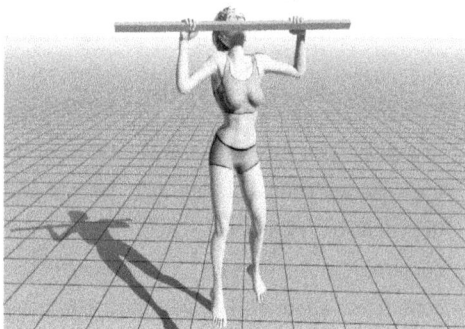

BACK ROW WITH TOWEL, ROPE OR BELT- Option 2

The Lower back row is a great exercise for developing the back muscles. ISO Row: Take a seat and bend your legs so you can reach and choke up on the towel. Pull the towel towards you and keep your shoulders down and away from your ears; this will allow you to not only feel your arms but also the lats and rear deltoids. Hold for 6-8 sec, relax for 2-3 seconds and repeat. You should be contracting about 80% of your max effort. Do 10 repetitions.

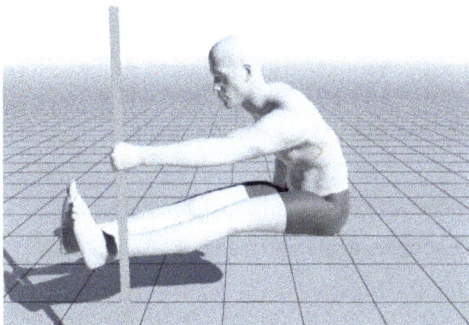

THE SCAPULAR HOLD

The Scapular Hold is one of the most important exercises in this program. It helps improve joint functionality while alleviating aches and pains that may come from sitting behind a desk. Prolonged sitting leaves the upper and lower back and glutes inactive, which can cause them to become weak. Weakness in this area can cause a forward tilt, which leads to more stress on the lower spine. The Scapular Hold helps prevent this misalignment.

Lie on your back with your knees bent and your feet flat on the floor. Place your arms out by your sides at a 45-degree angle.

Bend your elbows so your forearms form a 90-degree angle with the floor.

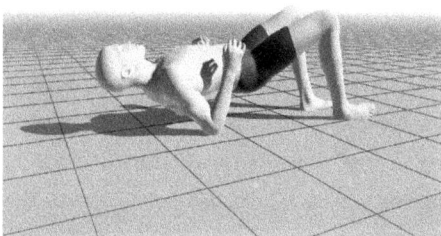

Squeeze your shoulder blades together and drive through your elbows and heels to lift your hips off the floor.

At the highest position, form a straight line from the back of your shoulders to the back of your knees. Pause.

Carefully lower back down.

LAT PULL USING YOUR KNEE

POSITION A: Sit erect on a chair. Bring your right knee up, with your right foot about 12" off the floor. Clasp both hands around your right knee, interlocking the fingers and keeping your arms straight. Now endeavor to pull your right knee back while resisting the effort with your right leg. Slowly intensify the effort while inhaling 3 to 4 seconds until you reach peak contraction. Begin a slowly controlled exhalation for 7 to 12 seconds while making an f-f-f-f or s-s-s-s sound and maintaining the intensity of the contraction the entire time. Then slowly release the tension as you inhale for 3 to 4 seconds. Relax. Power breathe for 7 to 10 reps and then repeat the entire procedure on the left side.

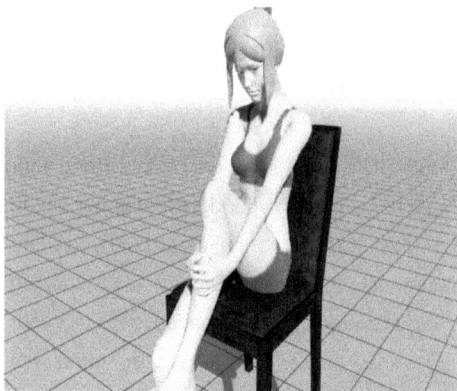

LOWER BACK BRIDGE

GLUTE BRIDGE

Lie face-up on the floor with your knees up at 90 degrees and your feet flat on the floor, shoulder-width apart. Tilt your pelvis back so you scoop the tailbone under, and then squeeze your glutes to lift the hip bones up into the air. Hold this position and breathe. Start with a shorter duration of 20 seconds and build your way up to a full minute.

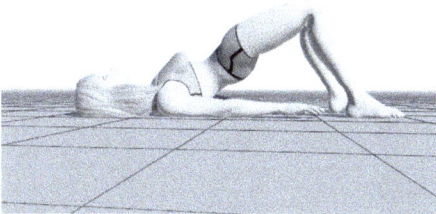

CHEST WITHOUT EQUIPMENT

PUSH UP HOLD (HALF WAY)

Isometric push-up hold

Place your hands directly under your shoulders and extend your arms to begin. Assure you have a neutral spine from head to feet. Engage your midsection and core as you bend your elbows and descend your chest to the floor. Stop the descent when your elbows reach 90 degrees and HOLD this position isometrically.

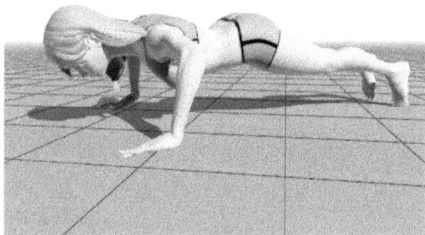

CHEST SQUEEZE
INTERLOCKED FINGERS/PUSHING PALMS
TOGETHER

ISOMETRIC CHEST SQUEEZE
Place your palms together in front of the chest as if you're praying, and then press them together tightly by squeezing your chest and shoulder muscles. Hold for 20-60 seconds at a time and remember to breathe. You can change the position of your hands to be higher or lower and closer to the chest or farther away in order to increase or decrease the difficulty of the movement.

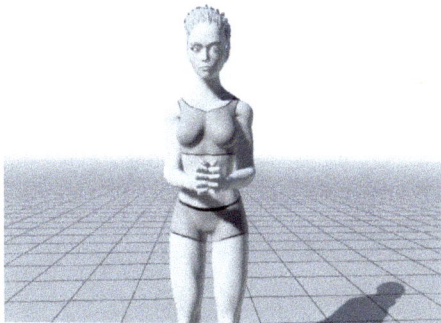

WALL PUSHUP HOLD

Start facing the wall approximately 18 inches away; lean in and place hands on the wall at chest height, shoulder-width apart. Slowly lower your body in towards the wall by bending your arms. Stop once your arms are at the midway point or 90 degrees. Hold that position for 10 seconds. Don't forget to breathe.

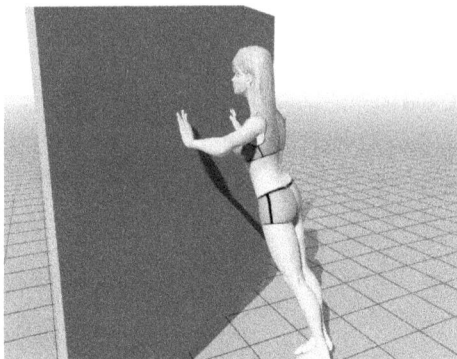

SHOULDERS WITH SMALL WEIGHT (5 or 10 pounds) OR ROPE

SIDE LATERAL RAISE

To execute, slowly raise the dumbbells up to around shoulder height. It's important that you do not let your wrists go above your elbows while raising the weight, as this will take the work off the side deltoids and put it on the front deltoids.

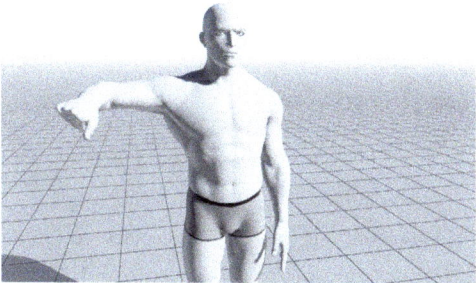

Against the wall

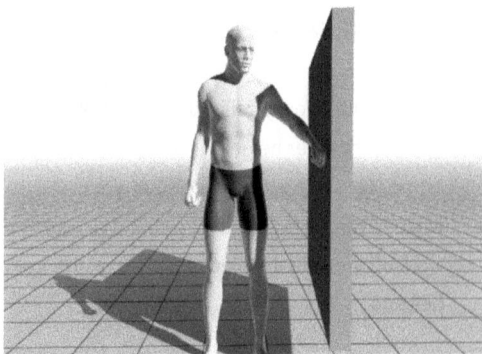

PIKE PUSH UP/ ELEVATED FEET

Start in a plank position on the floor, with hands firmly on the floor, right under your shoulders. Lift your legs and place your toes on elevated surface. Keep the core tight and back flat and engage your glutes and hamstrings. Your whole body should be neutral and in a straight line.

Lift hips up and back until your body forms an inverted V shape. Keep arms and legs as straight as possible.
Start to bend your elbows, and then lower your entire upper body toward the floor.

Stay there for a moment, then slowly push back up until your arms are straight and you're in the inverted V position. Make sure you maintain control throughout the movement.

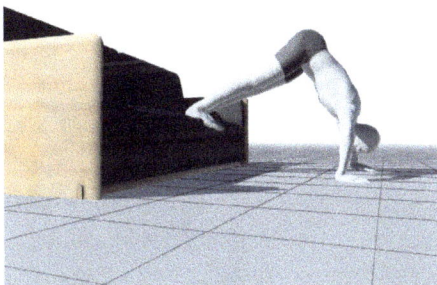

****The pike push-up is not a move for beginners, NOT recommended for anyone who's recovering from an elbow or shoulder injury.

PIKE PUSH UP -Not Elevated

Start in a plank position on the floor, with hands firmly on the floor, right under your shoulders. Press your toes firmly into the floor too.

Keep the core tight and back flat and engage your glutes and hamstrings. Your whole body should be neutral and in a straight line.

Lift hips up and back until your body forms an inverted V shape. Keep arms and legs as straight as possible.

Start to bend your elbows, and then lower your entire upper body toward the floor.

Stay there for a moment, then slowly push back up until your arms are straight and you're in the inverted V position. Make sure you maintain control throughout the movement.

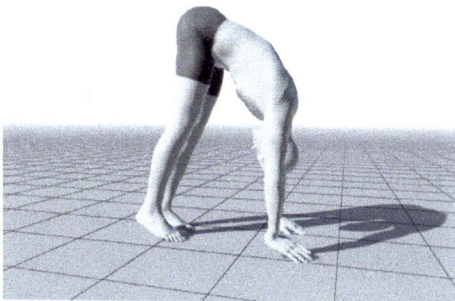

FRONT LATERAL RAISE

Raise arms to side, Elbows bent slightly. Lift to shoulder height (Not above 90 degrees). Holding a weight, rope or belt tied to something. Continue with the opposite arm. Or do both arms at the same time.

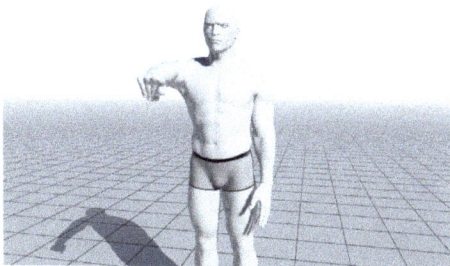

BENT OVER REAR DELTOID RAISE

Upper body bent over, raise upper arms to sides until elbows are shoulder height. Maintain upper arms perpendicular to torso and fixed elbow position (10° to 30° angle) throughout exercise.

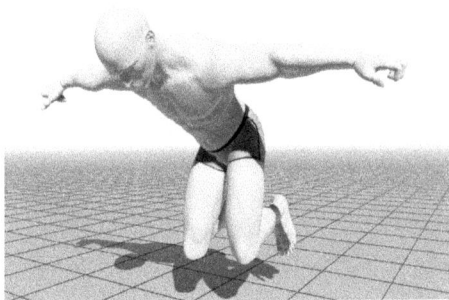

SHOULDER DOORWAY PRESS

SHOULDERS
WITHOUT EQUIPMENT
DOORWAY, CEILING PRESS/WALL
LATERAL RAISE

Stand in a door frame
lift the arms and bring your hands shoulder
width against the horizontal part of the door
frame. Press up and hold with as much force
as you can stand

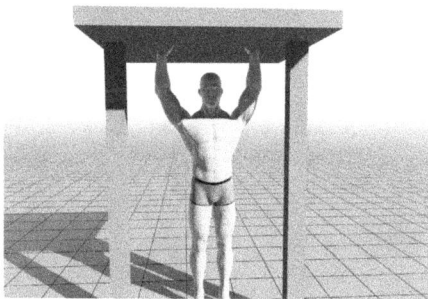

TRAP SHRUG WITH WEIGHT

With your hands under the back of your thighs, Slowly "shrug" until your traps will be fully contracted (flexed). Keep your legs locked straight. You are using the resistance to do the shrug. Think of it as trying to touch your shoulders to your ears. Then slowly lower your shoulders until the bar is back in the starting position. Remember to keep your arms straight and look forward throughout the set. You can sit grabbing under your thigh, pull up and shrug.

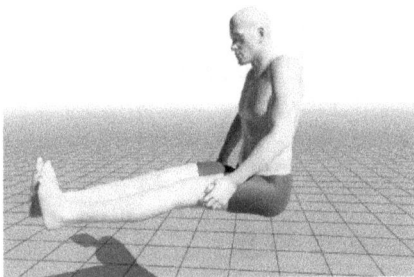

NECK exercises

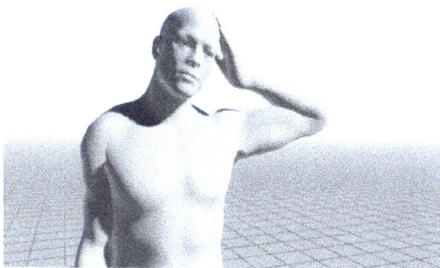

Side

Press Neck into your hand. Lock arm and hand so it does not move. Hold the press for 10 seconds, switch sides.

Front

Press Neck forward into your hand. Lock arm
and hand. Hold press for 10 seconds.

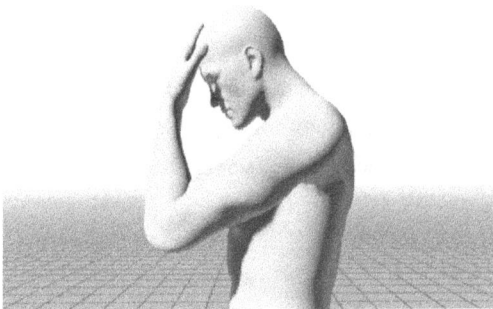

Back

Press Neck back into your hand. Lock arm and hand. Hold press for 10 seconds.

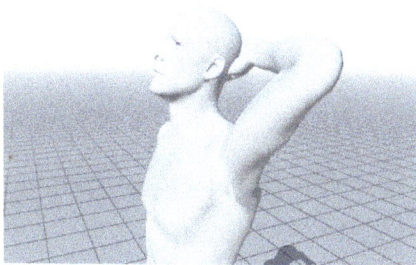

BICEPS WITHOUT EQUIPMENT

BICEP CURL

Bend your right arm at a 90-degree angle.
Grab your right hand with your left hand. Push
them together as hard as you can. While your
left biceps prevents your arm from dropping,
your right triceps is trying to push your right
arm down. 10 second hold. Repeat on the
other side.

Bicep Curl against opposite hand

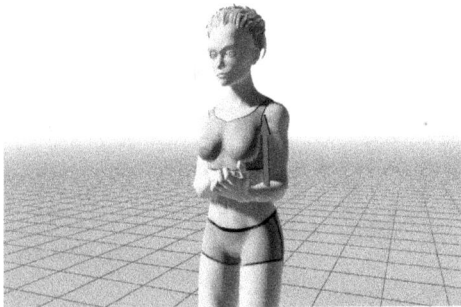

BICEP WITH BAR, TOWEL OR ROPE

Start standing with a dumbbell in each hand. Your elbows should rest at your sides and your forearms should extend out in front of your body. ...

Anchor towel or rope to heavy object or stand on rope/towel. Bring the dumbbells all the way up to your shoulders by bending your elbows. Once at the top, hold for 10 seconds by squeezing the muscle. At a 90-degree angle.

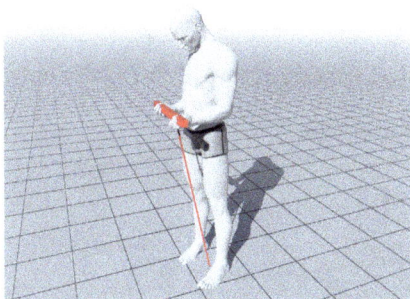

TRICEPS WITHOUT EQUIPMENT

Get into a lunge position with your fists on the wall at head level. Use your triceps to push your fists into the wall.Hold there, then return to an upright position.

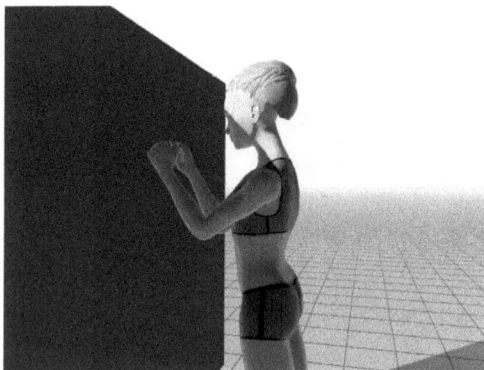

CLOSE GRIP TRICEP HOLD

Lower toro while hands are close together. Once arms are at 90 degrees Hold for 10 seconds.Hold at the top and bottom. When you have mastered the top and bottom add in a hole in the middle, halfway down.

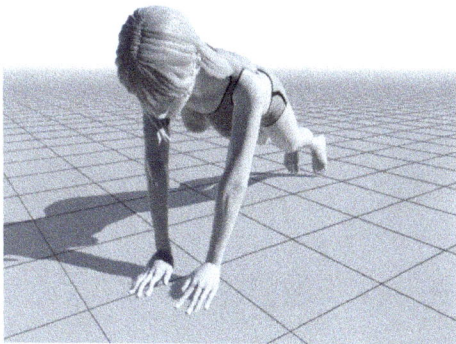

TRICEP PRESS DOWN AGAINST KNEE

Press Down with both hands, concentrate on the tricep and how it is being worked. Hold for 10 seconds.

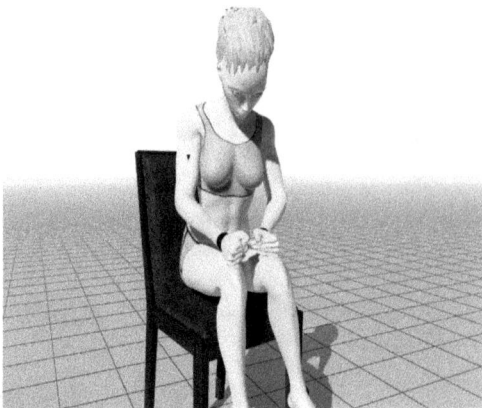

TRICEP DIP HOLD WITH CHAIR

Sit on the edge of the chair and grip the edge next to your hips. Your fingers should be pointed at your feet. Your legs are extended, and your feet should be about hip width apart with the heels touching the ground. Look straight ahead with your chin up.

Press into your palms to lift your body and slide forward just far enough that your behind clears the edge of the chair.

Lower yourself until your elbows are bent between 45 and 90 degrees.

HOLD there for a count of 10 seconds.

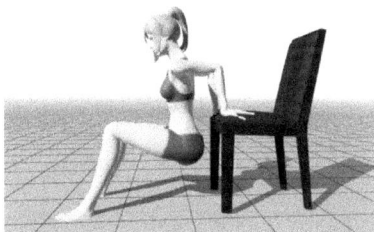

TRICEP EXTENSION WITH TOWEL, ROPE OR BELT

Start off standing with your feet shoulder width apart, your back straight and your abs drawn in.

Hold a towel or rope facing up behind and in back of your head.

Lower your forearms down until it's at around 90 degrees. Then slowly raise your arm back up to starting position while pulling down with the other hand on the towel.

Grasp the rope with a neutral grip (palms facing in) and lean forward slightly by hinging at the hips.

Initiate the movement by extending the elbows and flexing the triceps.

Pull the rope downward until the elbows are at 90 degrees, HOLD for 10 seconds

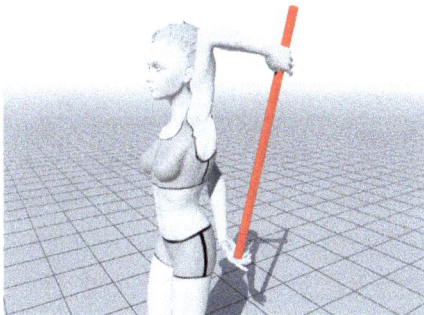

BI/TRI COMBO

Stand erect with your feet about 12" apart. Clench both fists as tightly as possible and place them as shown with your left fist over your right at close to full extension.

With your right arm pulling up and your left arm pressing down, slowly build tension in both arms while inhaling for 3 to 4 seconds until you reach maximum contraction. Hold this maximum contraction for 7 to 12 seconds, slowly exhaling and making an f-f-f-f or SSSSSS sound. Then slowly release the tension for another 3 to 4 seconds while inhaling slowly. Relax. Power breathe, then switch arms to right over left, following the exact same breathing and contraction procedures outlined above.

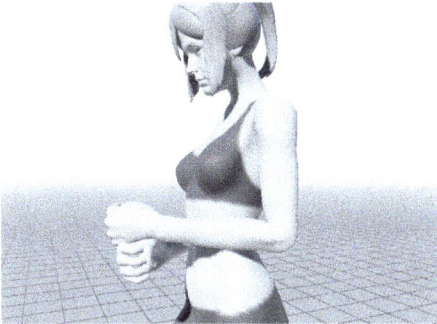

ABS

Lie on the floor with your feet together and
toes pointed forward and down. Arms by your
side Now raise your head and shoulders off
the ground and endeavor to touch your chin to
your chest as you inhale for 3 to 4 seconds
while trying to sit up against the powerful
resistance provided by your hands.

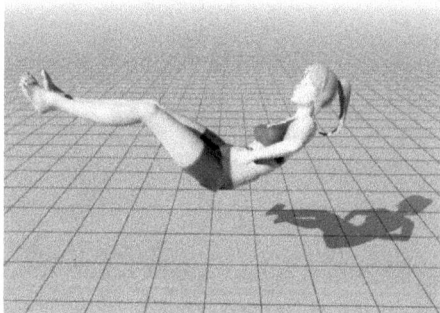

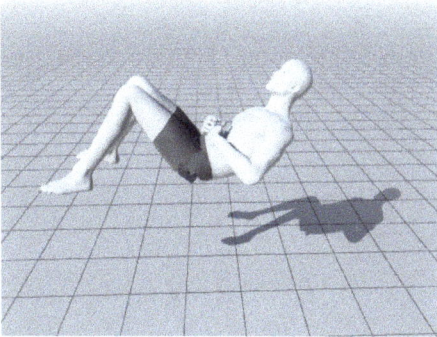

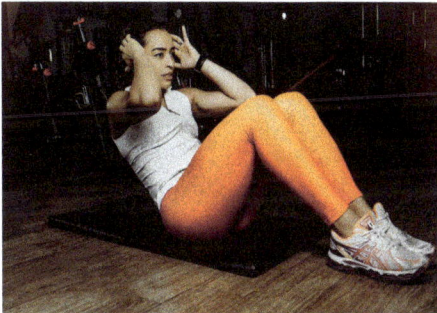

STATIC HOLD ARM ANGLES- 5 POSITION
HOLD

This is an exercise you can do after you have mastered the single or two position hold.

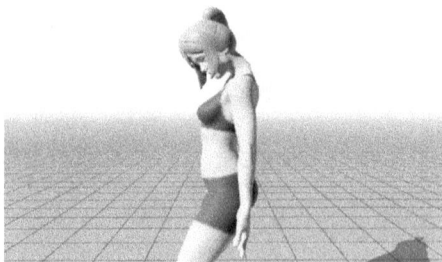

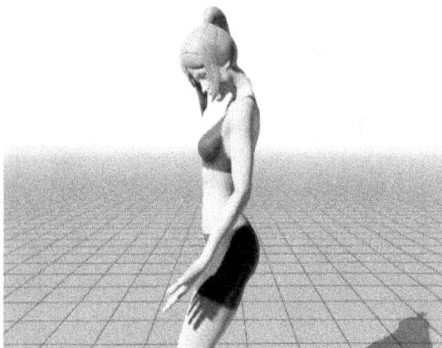

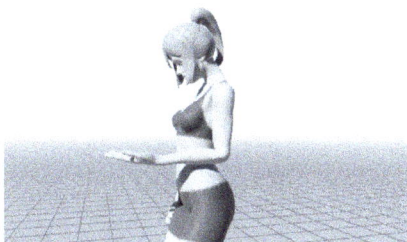

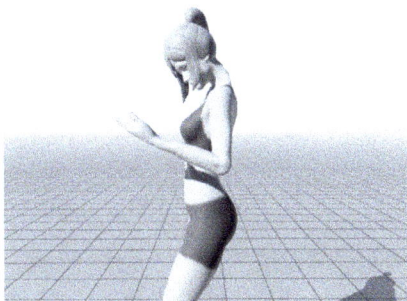

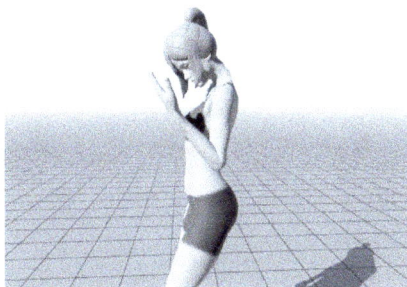

171

BUILD YOUR OWN BOD

As with any workout program once you get comfortable you always look to enhance your workouts. Hysometrics Builds strength. You can utilize that strength to enhance certain muscle groups to your liking. For example, some men think that having big arms or a thick chest is impressive. Women like to have tight legs and strong butt muscles. The Muscle groups below show you what groups pertain to your body.

No Individual is the same.

Exercises that build thick shoulders on one person may not work at all on another. It becomes experimentation. This is Exactly why I encourage you all to keep a log of your workouts. Refer to them every couple of weeks to analyze your progress. This is a BIG part of using your mind to build your body. HYSOMETRICS takes a cerebral approach to reaching your goals. Research, take notes and learn as much as you can about what works and doesn't work for you!

Legs

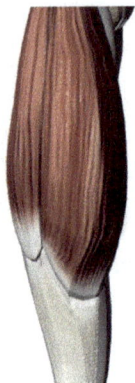

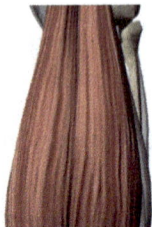

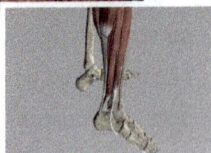

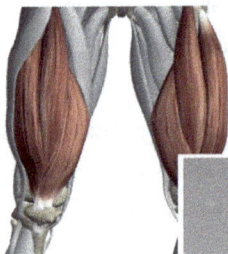

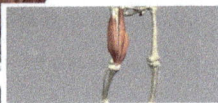

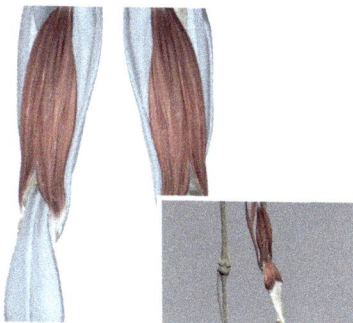

Back

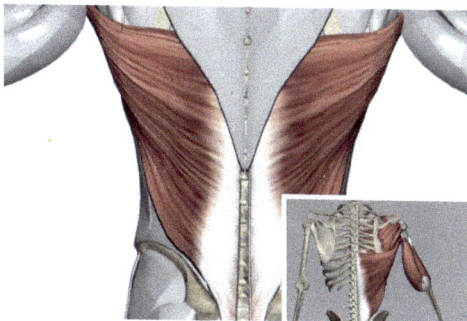

Chest

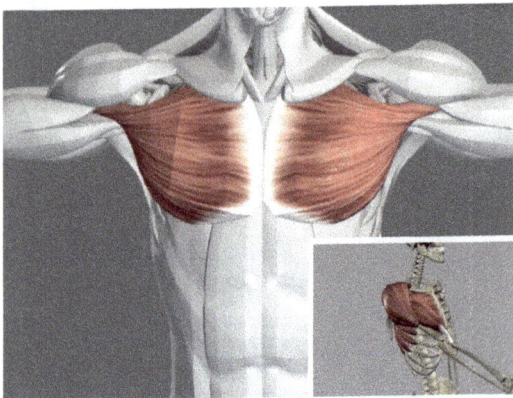

Shoulders

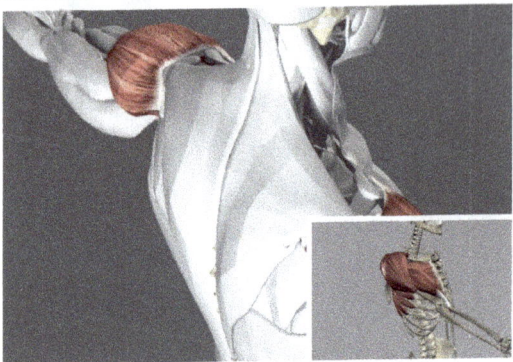

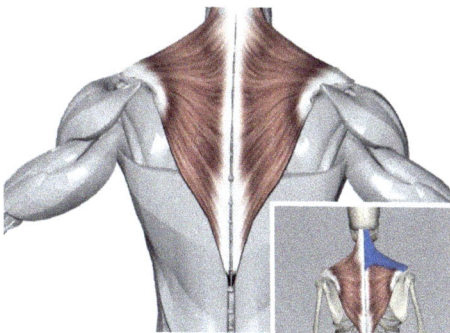

Traps

Neck

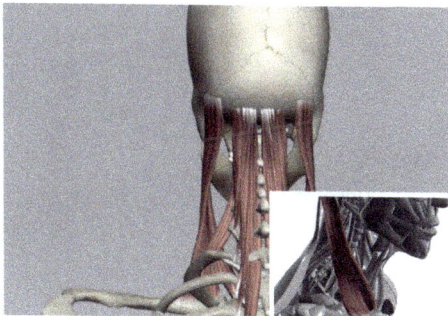

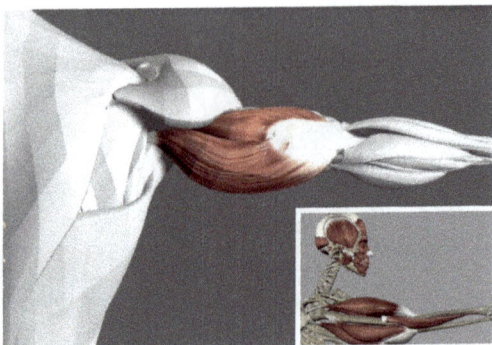

Triceps
Biceps

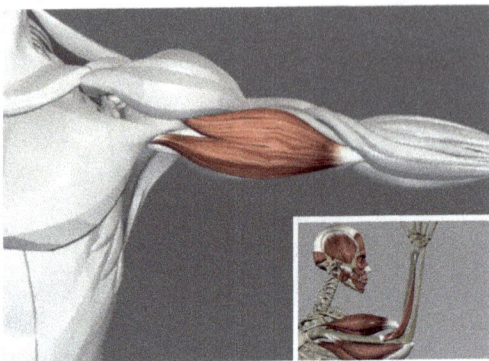

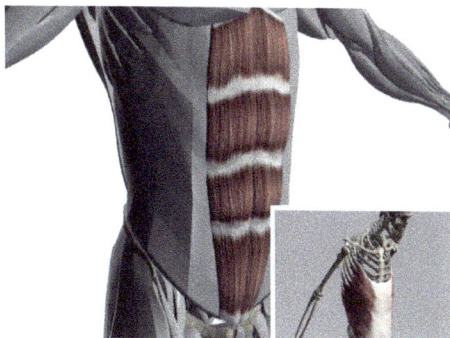

Abs

'SUPER SET' EXAMPLE:

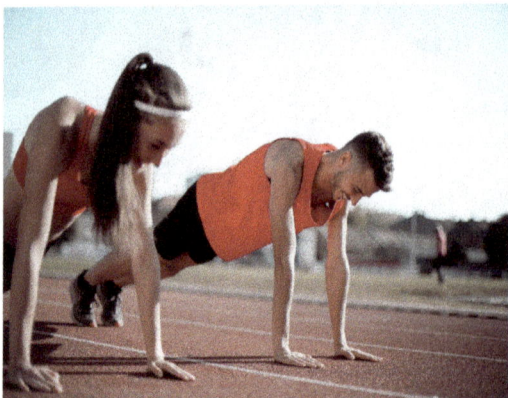

CHEST

Super Set. 2 Exercises performed back-to-back with NO REST in between.

1. **ISOMETRIC HOLD**
2. **DYNAMIC MOVEMENT**

EXAMPLE: HYSOMETRIC SUPER SET
ISOMETRIC & ISO-BOW, DUMBBELL or BAND

SET 1

ISOMETRIC CHEST PUSH HOLD (HALFWAY) 10 SECONDS

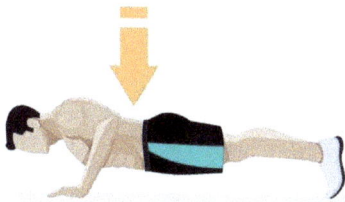

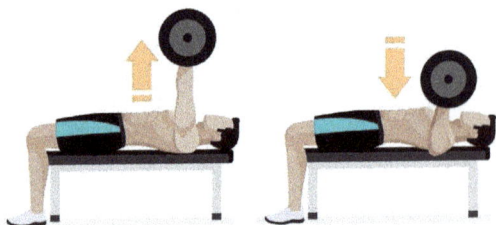

+

(Set 2)

DUMBBELL BENCH PRESS or WITH
BAND (10 Reps)

EXAMPLE: OF HYSOMETRIC 'SUPER SET' ISO & DUMBBELL

SET 1
1.WALL TRICEP HOLD 10 SECONDS

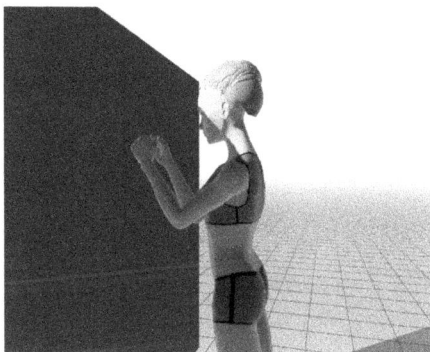

2. Dumbbell Tricep Extension

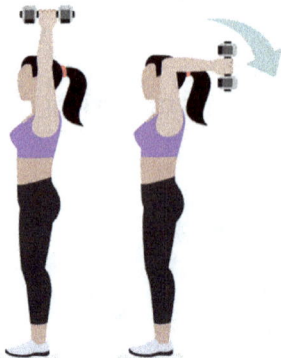

REST 30 seconds
Repeat sets 1 & 2
Rest 30 seconds
Repeat sets 1 & 2
Rest 30 seconds onto next body part

BREAKDOWN:

BASIC HYSOMETRIC WORKOUT FORMULA

Set 1 (ISOMETRIC 10 second hold)
Set 2 (DYNAMIC SET- 10 REPS)
Rest 30 seconds
Repeat
Rest 30 seconds
Repeat
Rest 30 second onto next body part

FULL BODY workout:

(3 sets) CONSISTING OF

1 ISOMETRIC SET &
1 DYNAMIC SET
Superset (back-to-back)

LEGS

CALF's

BACK

CHEST

SHOULDERS

TRAPS

NECK

TRICEPS

BICEPS

A workout superset is a training
technique in which two exercises are
performed back-to-back without rest in
between. The two exercises in a
superset are typically chosen to target

different muscle groups or movement patterns, allowing for efficient and time-saving workouts. The main concept behind super setting is to increase the intensity and challenge the muscles by working them in quick succession, effectively promoting muscle growth, endurance, and cardiovascular fitness.

Here's an example to illustrate how a superset works:

Select two exercises that target different muscle groups. Let's say you choose push-ups (chest, triceps, shoulders) and squats (quadriceps, glutes, hamstrings).

Begin by performing a set of push-ups until you reach muscle fatigue or a predetermined rep range. Immediately after completing the push-ups, without resting, move directly to the squat exercise.

Perform a set of squats until you reach muscle fatigue or the desired rep range.

Rest for a predetermined period, usually around 30-90 seconds.

Repeat the superset for the desired number of sets.
The key benefits of incorporating supersets into your workout routine include:

Time efficiency: Since you're performing two exercises in succession, you can complete a higher volume of work in less time compared to traditional sets with rest intervals.
Increased intensity: Supersets challenge your muscles by reducing the rest time, leading to increased muscle recruitment and metabolic stress.

Improved cardiovascular fitness: The continuous movement from one exercise to another without rest elevates your heart rate, providing a cardiovascular workout along with strength training.

Muscle conditioning and endurance: Supersets can enhance muscular endurance by pushing your muscles to work harder and adapt to the increased demands.

It's worth noting that there are different types of supersets, including compound supersets (two exercises targeting the same muscle group), opposing muscle group supersets (exercises targeting antagonist muscle groups), and upper/lower body supersets (one upper body exercise paired with one lower body exercise). The specific type of superset you choose depends on your fitness goals and the muscle groups you want to target.

NEVER, NEVER do the same pattern twice.

If you do let's say Push Upholds & Band Chest Press, the next chest workout you do a different order or even two different exercises. One of the Main principles of the HYSOMETRIC POWER PROGRAM is to NEVER do the same routine twice in a row. This will keep your mind and body from anticipating the next moves and work your muscles at different angles.

MOVEMENTS FOR BASIC DYNAMIC EXERCISE CHARTS

(Each exercise that utilizes weights
can be done with ISO-BOW,
dumbbells, or resistance bands)

3 sets × 12 reps

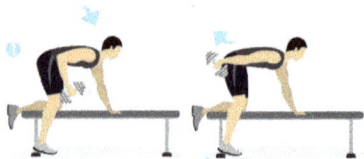

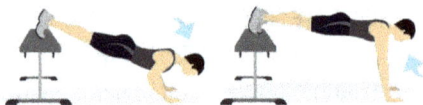

full plank 60 seconds

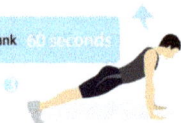

Elbow plank 60 seconds

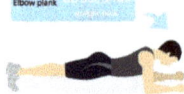

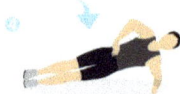

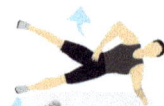

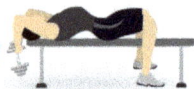

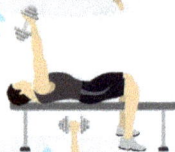

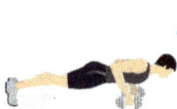

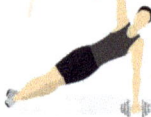

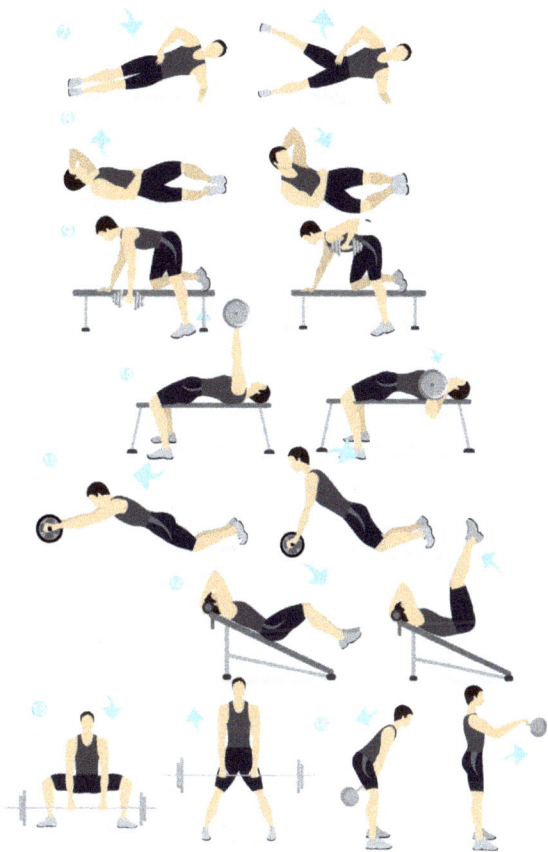

3 sets x 12 reps

194

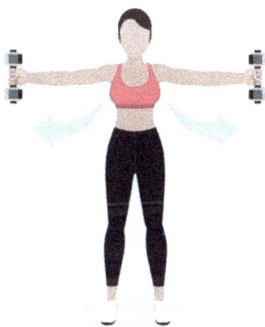

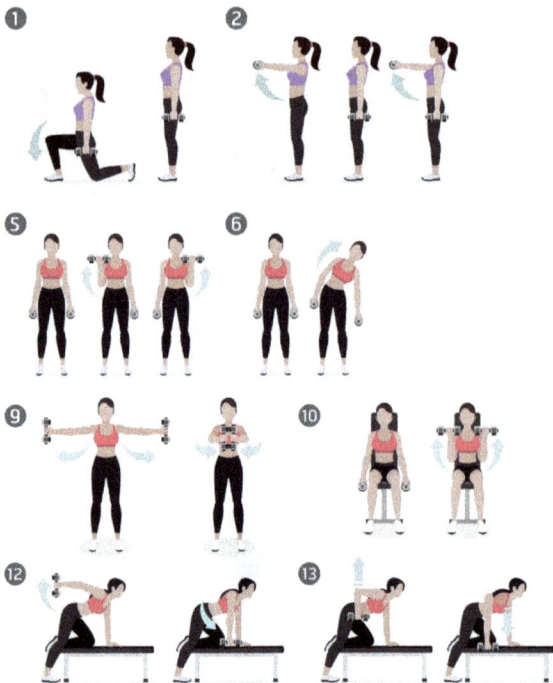

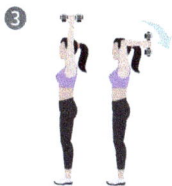

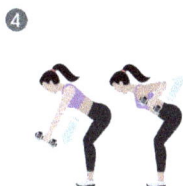

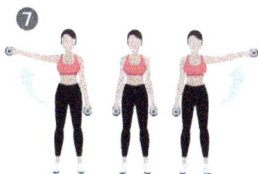

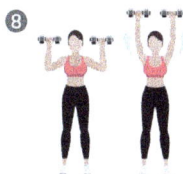

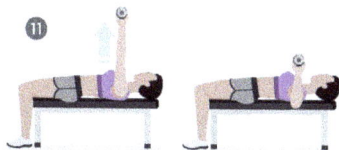

ISO QUICK STRENGTH

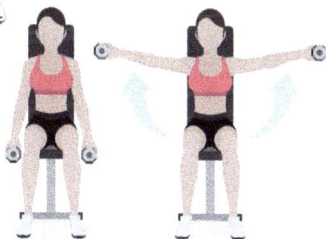

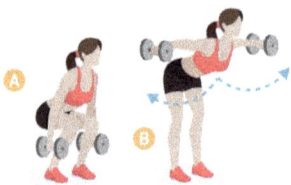

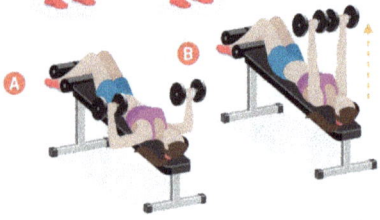

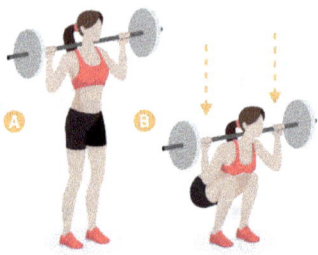

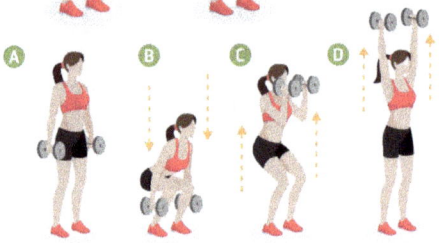

198

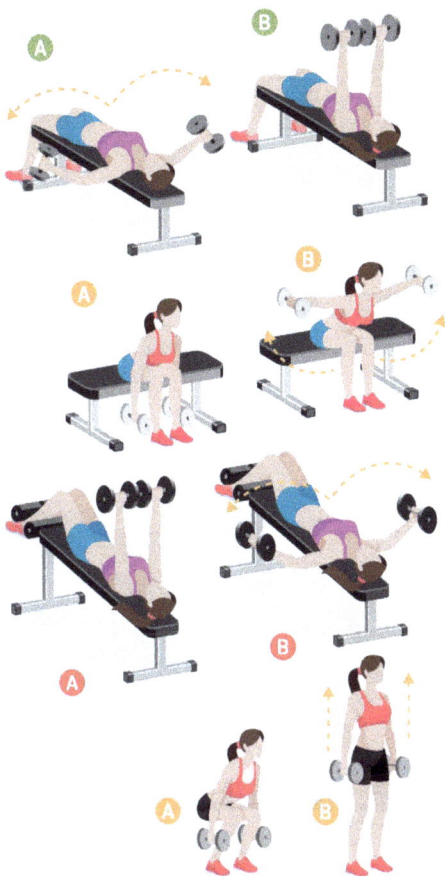

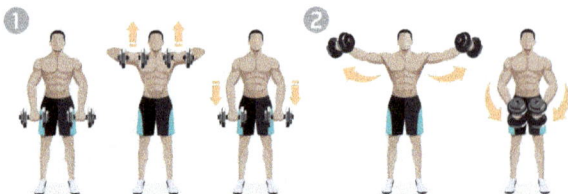

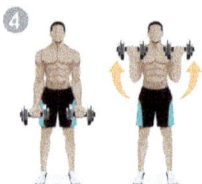

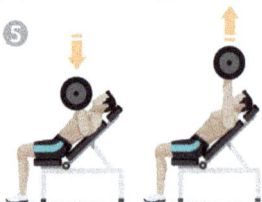

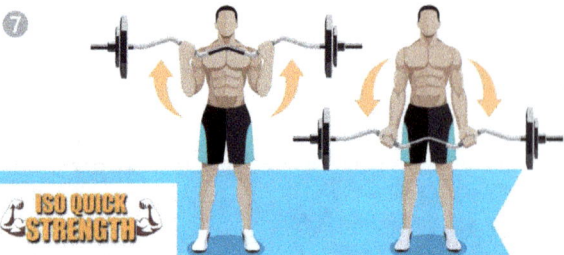

ISO QUICK STRENGTH

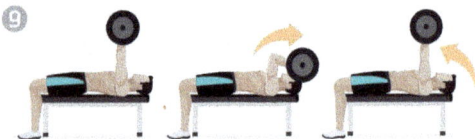

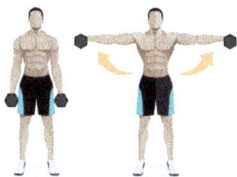

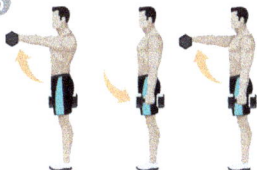

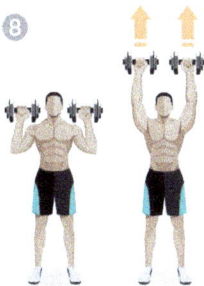

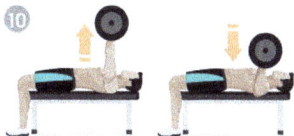

① 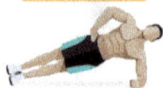 Hold 45 seconds
Repeat 3 times

② Hold 45 seconds
Repeat 3 times
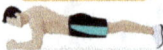

③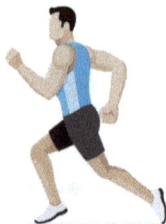

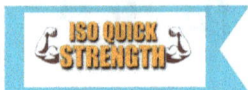 ISO QUICK STRENGTH ⑥

⑤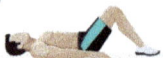

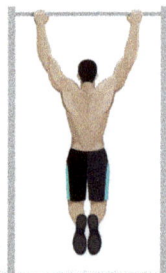

⑧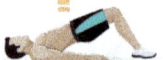

⑨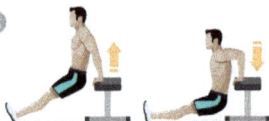

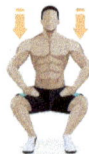

⑪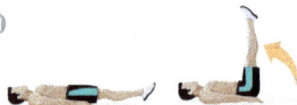

202

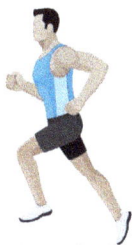
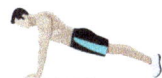
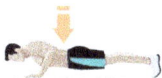
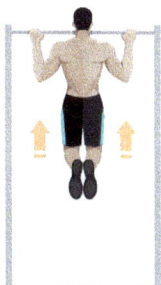
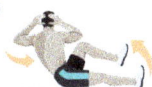
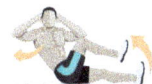
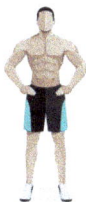
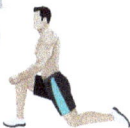
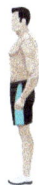
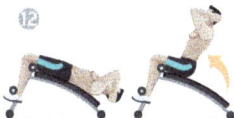

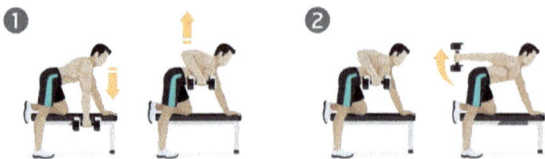

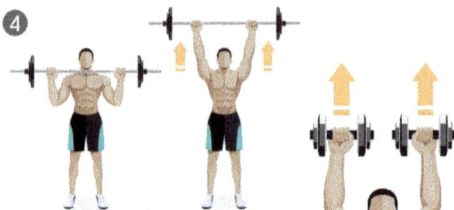

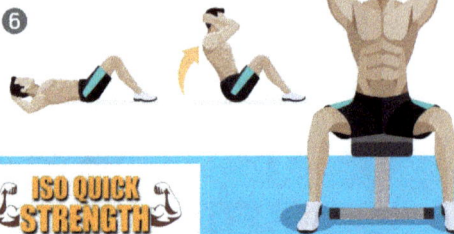

ISO QUICK STRENGTH

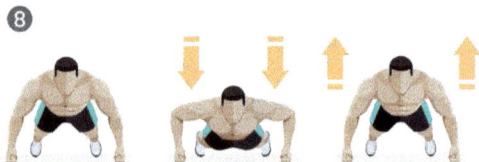

204

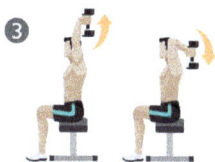

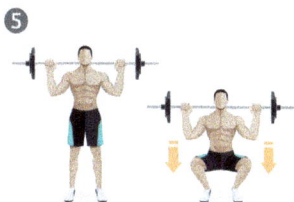

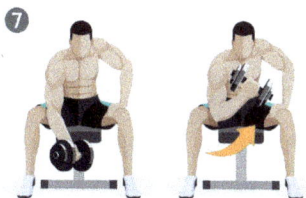

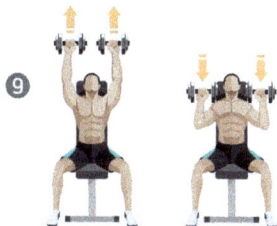

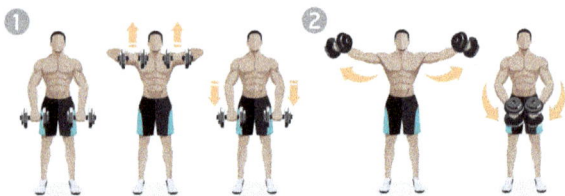

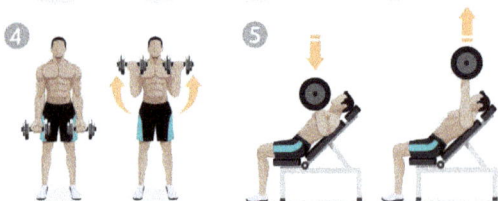

ISO QUICK STRENGTH

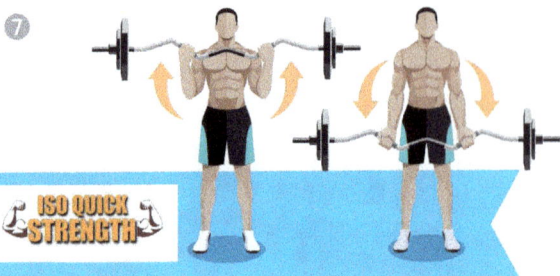

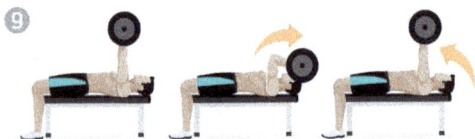

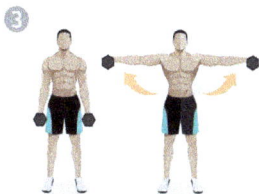

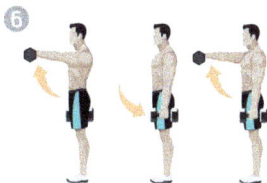

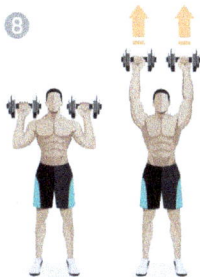

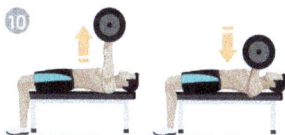

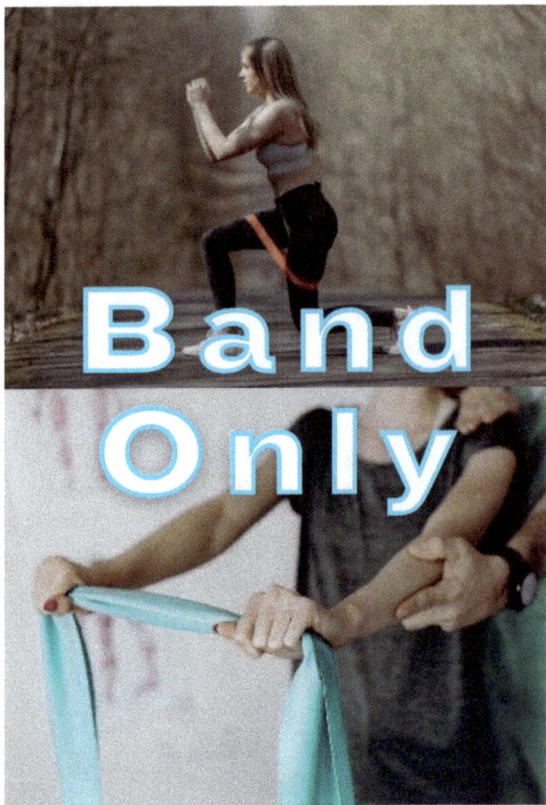

Band
Only

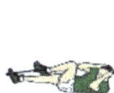
BICYCLE

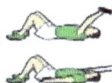
PULL OVER

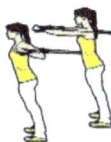
CHEST PRESS

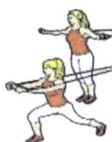
LUNGE FLY

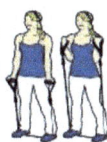
BICEP CURL LOW

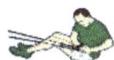
RUSSIAN TWIST

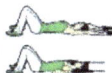
LAT PULL

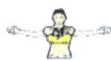
CHEST FLY

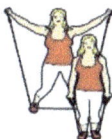
JUMPING JACKS

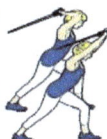
TRICEP EXTENSION

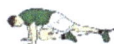
CROSS PLANK

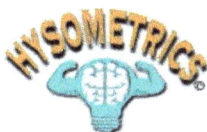

HYSOMETRICS

TRAIN THE MIND & BODY

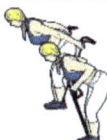
TRICEP KICKBACK

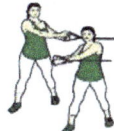
OBLIQUE TWIST

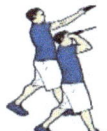
BICEP CURL HIGH

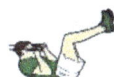
CRUNCHES

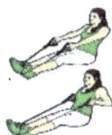
ROW

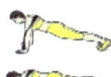
PUSH UP

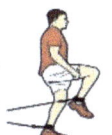
HIGH KNEES

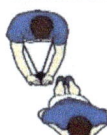
DIAMOND PU

209

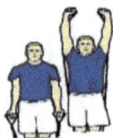
CURL PRESS

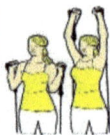
SHOULDER PRESS

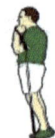
CALF RAISE

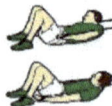
HEEL TOUCHES

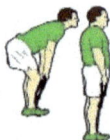
ROMANIAN DEADLIFT

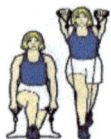
LUNGE FRONT RAISE

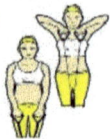
UPRIGHT ROWS

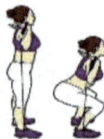
BACK SQUAT

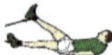
FLUTTER KICK

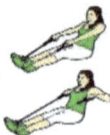
HIGH ROW

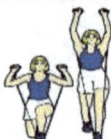
LUNGE PRESS

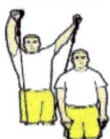
L RAISE

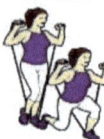
LUNGE

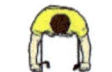
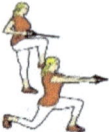
SPIDERMAN PU

LUNGE ROW KNEE

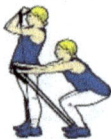
SQUAT CLEAN

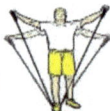
ARM CIRCLES

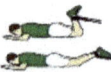
HAMSTRING CURL

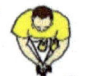
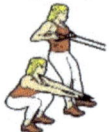
CLAP PUSH UP

SQUAT ROW

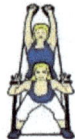
THRUSTER

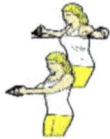
DELTOID FLY

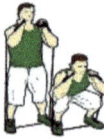
FRONT SQUAT

210

ISO QUICK STRENGTH

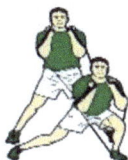

SIDE SQUAT

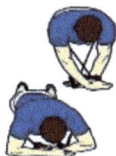

X ARM EXTENSION

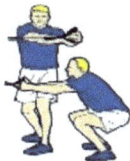

SQUAT TWIST

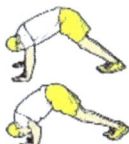

PIKE PUSH UP

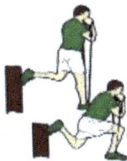

SPLIT SQUAT

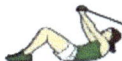

NO ROTATION CRUNCH

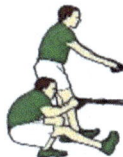

PISTOL SQUAT

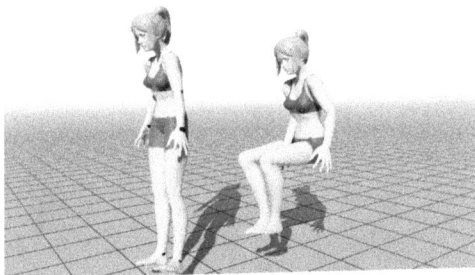

(Body weight) Wall Squat

(With weight) Dumbbell Row

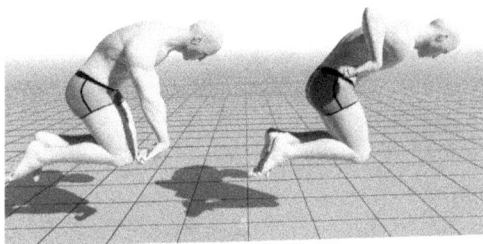

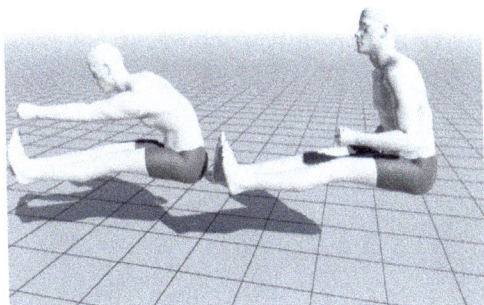

(Band) Band Seat Row

(Body weight) Push Up

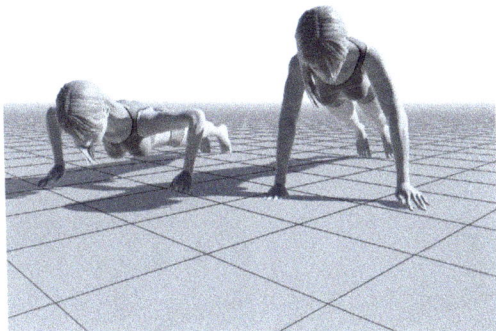

(With weight) Bench Press

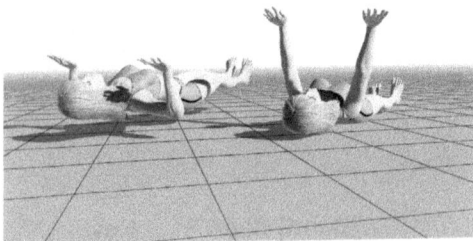

(With weight or band) Lateral Side Raise

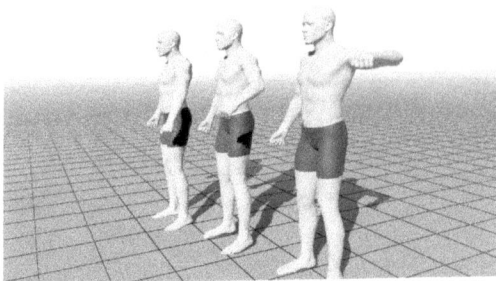

(With weight or band) Shoulder Press

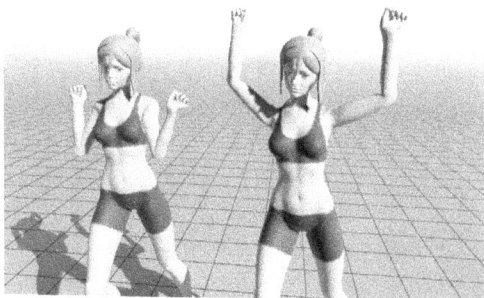

(Band) Band Tricep Pushdown

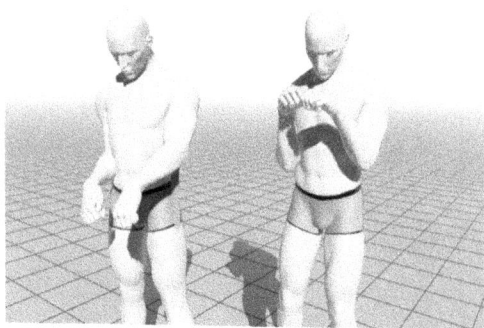

(With weight or band) Tricep Extension

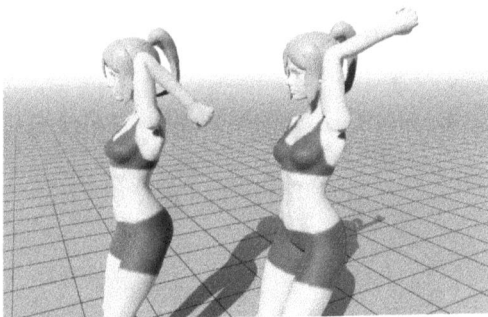

(Body weight) Tricep Wall Push

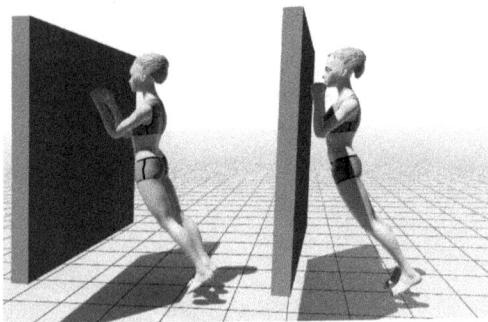

(With weight or band) Bicep Curl

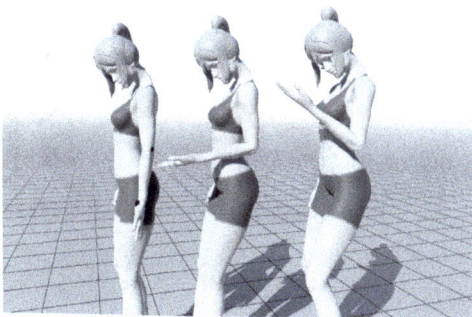

AB Crunches

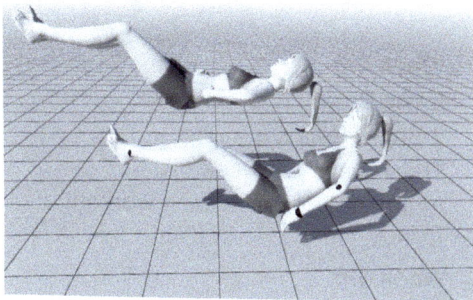

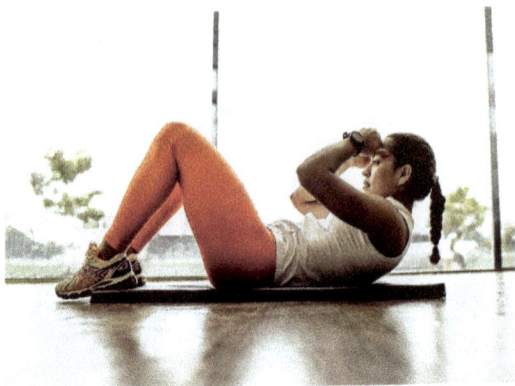

THE WORKOUT:

Keep a log for each and every workout
for 6-week evaluation.

Week 1-3
Basic Program for 3 weeks
2 Super Sets x 3
Three Days per week
Alternate Exercises each workout

Week 3-6
Step Up- 2 Super Sets x 4

Three Days per week
Alternate Exercises each workout

6 Week Evaluation.

'RAPID REPS' POWER-LIFT
(without the gym)

The 'Rapid Rep' concept is VERY simple. Powerlifter workouts are done with HEAVY weight usually Low reps maybe 1 or 2 reps.

Using **OVERCOMING ISOMETRICS** we are going to trick the mind into thinking that you are in fact benching 300 pounds. While Overcoming Isometrics has been around a long time, it's not as glamorous as lifting weights in a gym full of pretty people. Overcoming Isometrics was used by ALL the old time Strongmen. People that could lift cars, tear telephone phone books and bend steel bars.

Overcoming **isometrics is the act of attempting to lift or move an immovable object.**

Overcoming isometrics transfers a greater amount of energy to concentric strength and thereby demands more from the neurological pathways. Such moves lend themselves to short, intense efforts. This approach does not result in muscle damage and therefore cultivates much more **muscular strength** versus size.

The concept of Powerlifting is not for everyone. The average person wants to just tone their muscles and keep their weight down. However, lifting heavy weights for low reps is for those that wish to or need to become strong for their jobs, lifestyle or just to survive the daily rigors of life.

So how does it work you ask?

Simple. You find something that is considered **IMMOVABLE**, try moving it while your brain, your body and all your nerves fire to accomplish the task.

In Powerlifting you would find that 1 rep max and attempt to complete the lift. Be it bench press, squat, deadlift etc... With a 'RAPID REP' you will use a chain, rope, suspension strap or even a bar against the racks pins to attempt the lift.

It has been said that OVERCOMING ISOMETRICS is only limited by how hard you exert. For this movement we are going at 100%, EVERYTHING you have for 4 seconds. Why four seconds? **The average power-lift rep takes**

between 4 and 6 seconds depending on how hard and heavy the weight is.

As in powerlifting, you will take your 4 second rep, then rest 30- 60 seconds before doing a second. I ask that you attempt 5, 4 second reps with rest in between.

Big Inhale at the beginning, big exhale as you push.

The MOVEMENT is a BURST of strength, 100% effort.
Holding against the object for 4 full seconds
then resting.

The mind does not know the difference between the chain tied to the bumper of your truck or an Olympic bar loaded with six 45-pound plates.

All the brain wants to do is satisfy you by making the lift. It will call in all its resources to do so. And the beauty of Isometrics is that it will also call in the nerve receptors to help if it can. I can tell you that this is not only hard, but also Exhausting!

You will have to get VERY creative if you don't have a well-stocked weight room. I like to use chains and suspension straps, or tow straps connected to my bench. Chains will NEVER break.

Example using a bench against the bar holder

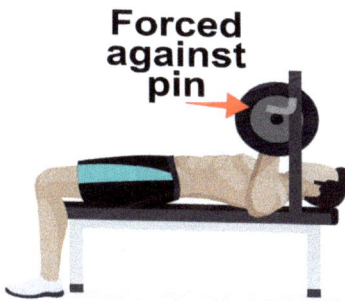

Forced against pin

If you are using a Chain or Suspension/Tow strap simple wrap under the bench and adjust to the proper length.

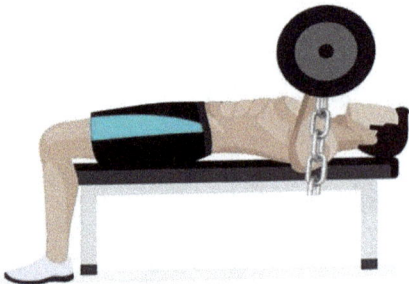

Other examples with chain, suspension or tow strap anchored:

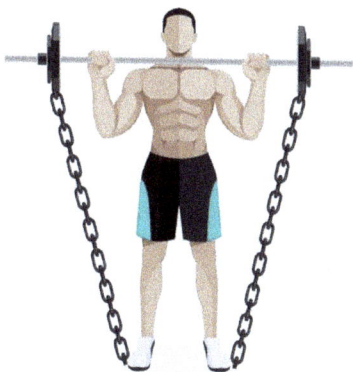

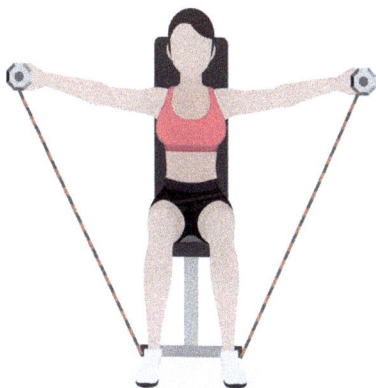

225

Squat with Strap/Chain

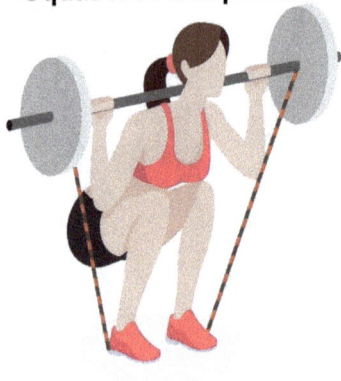

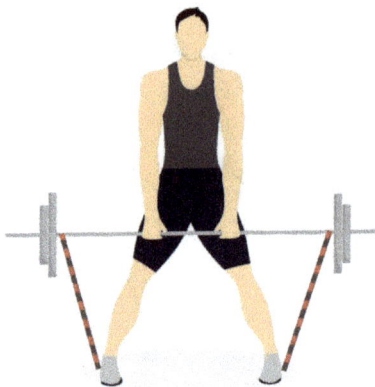

SAMPLE WORKOUT LOG

Date:	Weight:		Cardio:					
Exercise:	Reps	Weight	Reps	Weight	Reps	Weight	Reps	Weight

Date:	Weight:		Cardio:					
Exercise:	Reps	Weight	Reps	Weight	Reps	Weight	Reps	Weight

Date:	Weight:		Cardio:					
Exercise:	Reps	Weight	Reps	Weight	Reps	Weight	Reps	Weight

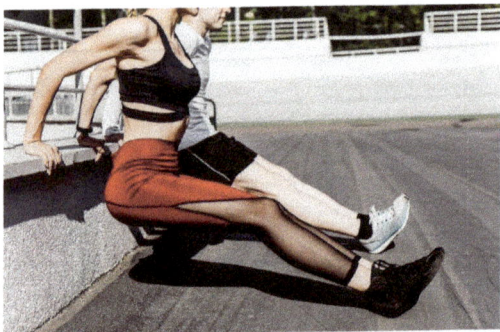

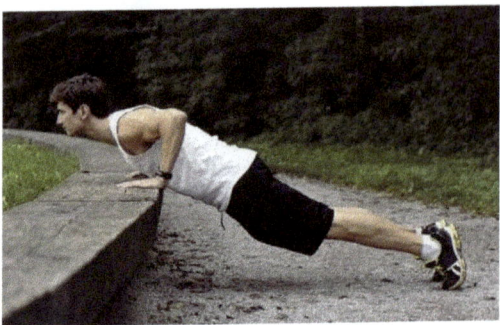

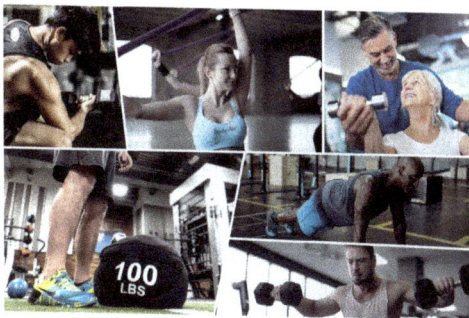

FITNESS TERMINOLOGY

Activities of Daily Living (ADLs)- Physical tasks of everyday living, such as bathing, and walking up the stairs. ADLs are usually factored into a person's basal metabolic rate, so tracking calories burned for these types of movement isn't recommended when trying to lose weight.

Aerobic exercise- Any rhythmic activity that increases the body's need for oxygen by using large muscle groups continuously for at least

10 minutes. The term aerobic means "with oxygen."

Agonist muscle- A muscle that is highly effective in causing a certain joint movement. Also called the prime mover. On a biceps curl, the biceps are the agonist muscle that flexes the elbow joint.

Amenorrhea- The absence of menstruation, commonly found in women with an exceptionally low body fat percentage and/or exercise excessively.

Anaerobic exercise- Short lasting, high intensity activity, where the demand for oxygen from the exercise exceeds the oxygen supply.

Angina pectoris- Chest pain due to lack of blood flow (oxygen) to the heart.

Antagonist muscle- A muscle that causes movement at a joint in a direction opposite to that of the joint's agonist (prime mover).

Beta-blockers- Type of medication that reduces heart rate. Exercisers who take beta-blockers will have a lower heart rate at rest and during exercise, so the target heart rate formula cannot be used in this case.

Bioelectrical impedance- This method of measuring body composition is because the lean tissue of the body is much more conductive due to its higher water content than fat tissue. The leaner tissue present in the body, the greater the conductive potential, measured in ohms.

Body composition- Amount of fat vs. lean muscle tissue in the human body.

Body Mass Index (BMI)- Measure of the relationship between height and weight;

calculated by dividing weight in kilograms by height in centimeters squared.

Caffeine- A stimulant found in coffee, tea, chocolate, and some soft drinks that increases heart contractions, oxygen consumption, metabolism, and urinary output.

Calisthenics- Exercising using one's own body weight which helps develop muscular tone.

Cardiorespiratory fitness- Measure of the heart's ability to pump oxygen-rich blood to the muscles. Also called cardiovascular or aerobic fitness.

Cardiovascular system- A complex system consisting of the heart and blood vessels; transports nutrients, oxygen, and enzymes throughout the body and regulates temperature, water levels of cells, and acidity levels of body components.

Circuit training- Takes the participant through a series of exercise stations (which could also include strength training), with relatively brief rest intervals between each station. The purpose is to keep the heart rate elevated near the aerobic level without dropping off. The number of stations may range from 4 to 10.

Concentric muscle action- Force produced while the muscle is shortening in length.

Continuous training- This is the most common type of sustained aerobic exercise for fitness improvement, slowly adding more time to the workout to increase endurance.

Cool down- Lowering of body temperature following vigorous exercise. The practice of cooling down after exercise involves slowing down your level of activity gradually.

Core- A muscle group comprising the abdominals, lower back, obliques, and hips.

Cortisol- A hormone secreted by the adrenal gland that makes stored nutrients more readily available to meet energy demands. These hormone levels increase under stress, which can stimulate your appetite, leading to weight gain or difficulty losing weight.

Cross-training- An individualized combination of all aerobic-training methods, characterized by a variety of intensities and modes.

Detraining Principle- This principle says that once consistent exercise stops, you will eventually lose the strength that you built up. Without overload or maintenance, muscles will weaken in two weeks or less.

Diastolic blood pressure- The pressure exerted by the blood on the vessel walls during the resting portion of the cardiac cycle, measured in millimeters of mercury. Thediastolic number is the bottom of the fraction. 120/80 is the average value for normal blood pressure (80 is the diastolic number). Mild high blood pressure is between 140/90 and 160/95. High blood pressure is defined by a value greater than 160/95.

DOMS (Delayed Onset Muscle Soreness)- Muscle soreness or discomfort that appears 12 to 48 hours after exercise. It is most likely due to microscopic tears in the muscle tissue, and it usually requires a couple of days for the repair and rebuilding process to be completed. The muscle tissue grows back stronger, leading to increased muscle mass and strength.

Eccentric contraction- A lengthening of the muscle during its contraction; controls speed of movement caused by another force.

Ectomorph- A body shape characterized by a narrow chest, narrow shoulders and long, thin muscles.

Electrolytes- Salts (ions) found in bodily fluids. Pertaining to exercise, your body loses electrolytes (sodium, potassium) when you sweat. These electrolytes need to be replaced to keep concentrations constant in the body, which is why many sports drinks include electrolytes.

Endomorph- A body shape characterized by a round face, short neck, wide hips, and heavy fat storage.

Endorphins- Opiate-like hormones that are manufactured in the body and contribute to natural feelings of well-being.

EPOC (Excess Post-Exercise Oxygen Consumption)- This explains why your breathing rate remains heavy for a few minutes after finishing a workout. Your body needs more oxygen after a workout in order to restore the oxygen stores in the blood and tissues, and to meet the oxygen requirements of the heart rate, which is still elevated.

Epinephrine- Also called adrenaline, a hormone that stimulates body systems in response to stress.

Ergogenic aids- A substance, appliance, or procedure that improves athletic performance.

Eustress- "Good" stress that presents opportunities for personal growth. (Exercise is an example of this. It puts stress on the body and its systems, but the results of this stress are positive.)

Exercise metabolic rate (EMR)- The energy expenditure that occurs during exercise.
Fast twitch muscle fibers- Fibers that are better-suited for high-force, short duration

activities because they contain more stores for anaerobic energy utilization.

Fixed resistance- Strength training exercises that provide a constant amount of resistance throughout the full range of motion. Examples include free weights and resistance bands.
Flexibility- The measure of the range of motion, or the amount of movement possible, at a particular joint.

Graded Exercise Test (Incremental Exercise Test)- An exercise test involving a progressive increase in work rate over time. Often graded exercise tests are used to determine the subject's maximum oxygen consumption or lactic threshold.

Heart Rate Reserve (HRR)- Difference between resting and maximal heart rate.

Heat Cramps- Muscle cramps that occur during or following exercise in warm or hot weather.

Heat exhaustion- A heat stress illness caused by significant dehydration resulting from exercise in warm or hot conditions; frequent precursor to heat stroke.

Heat stroke- A deadly heat stress illness resulting from dehydration and overexertion in warm or hot conditions; can cause body core temperature to rise from normal to 100- or 105-degrees Fahrenheit in just a few minutes.

High-density lipoprotein (HDL)- Retrieves cholesterol from the body's cells and returns it to the liver to be metabolized. Also referred to as "good" cholesterol.

High impact- Activities that place more stress on the bones and joints, where your limbs are actually making contact with the ground or other surface with force. Examples include walking, running, step aerobics, and sports that involve impact, like basketball or tennis.

Hydrostatic (underwater) weighing- This method of measuring body composition is considered the "gold standard" and is based on the assumption that density and specific gravity of lean tissue is greater than that of fat tissue. By comparing the test subject's mass measured underwater and out of the water, body composition may be calculated.

Hyperplasia- An increase in the number of cells in a tissue; usually in reference to fat or muscle cells.

Hypertrophy- An increase in cell size (girth), usually in reference to fat or muscle cells.

Hypothermia- A life-threatening condition in which heat is lost from the body faster than it is produced.

Incremental Exercise Test (Graded Exercise Test)- An exercise test involving a progressive increase in work rate over time. Often these tests are used to determine the subject's maximum oxygen consumption or lactic threshold.

Interval training- Repeated intervals of exercise interspersed with intervals of relatively light exercise. This type of training provides a means of performing large amounts of high-intensity exercise in a short period of time.

Isokinetic exercise- Exercise in which the rate of movement is constantly maintained through a specific range of motion even though maximal force is exerted.

Isometric exercise- Any activity in which the muscles exert force but do not visibly change in length. For example, pushing against a wall or carrying a bag of groceries.

Isotonic exercise- Any activity in which the muscles exert force and change in length as they lift and lower resistance. For example, bicep curls or leg extensions.

Karvonen formula- One of the most effective methods used to calculate target heart rate. It factors resting heart rate into the equation.

Ketosis- A condition in which the body adapts to prolonged fasting or carbohydrate deprivation by converting body fat to ketones, which can be used as fuel for some brain activity. The real danger in ketosis is that ketones are acidic, and high levels of ketones make the blood abnormally acid.

Lactic acid- Once thought of as a waste substance that builds up in the muscles when they are not getting enough oxygen, leading to muscle fatigue and soreness. Now, experts believe that lactic acid is beneficial to the

242

body, acting as a "fuel" to help people continue high-intensity (anaerobic) exercise even when oxygen consumption is low.

Lactic threshold- The point at which the level of lactic acid in the blood suddenly increases (during exercise). This is a good indication of the highest sustainable work rate. Also known as anaerobic threshold.

Lean mass- Total weight of your muscle, bone, and all other body organs. (Everything in the body besides fat.)

Low-density lipoprotein (LDL)- Transports cholesterol and triglycerides from the liver to be used in various cellular processes. Also referred to as "bad" cholesterol.

Low impact- Activities that place less stress on the bones and joints. These are better for people with joint pain, and overweight individuals whose weight can hurt their joints.

Examples include swimming, elliptical, cycling, and other activities where your feet (or other body parts) aren't touching the ground with force or where you are somehow supported.

Max VO 2- (V02 Max) Highest amount of oxygen one can consume during exercise. The higher this number, the more you are cardiovascular fit and capable of increased levels of intensity.

Mesomorph- A body shape characterized by a large chest, long torso, solid muscle structure and significant strength.

MET- An expression of the energy it takes to sit quietly. It is frequently used as a measure of intensity on cardiovascular machines (treadmill, stationary bike, etc.) For example, moderate intensity activities are those that get you moving fast enough or strenuously enough to burn off three to six times as much energy per minute as you do when you are sitting quietly, measured as 3-6 METs.

Moderate intensity- Activities that range from 40-60% of max heart rate. These activities cause a slightly increased rate of breathing and feel light to somewhat hard. Individuals doing activity at this intensity can easily carry on a conversation.

Muscle fibers- Individual muscle cells that are the functional components of muscles.
Muscular endurance- The ability of the muscle to perform repetitive contractions over a prolonged period of time.

Muscular strength- The ability of the muscle to generate the maximum amount of force.
Obesity- A weight disorder generally defined as an accumulation of fat beyond that considered normal for a person based on age, sex, and body type.

One-Rep Max (1 RM)- The amount of weight/resistance that can be lifted or moved once, but not twice; a common measure of strength.

Opposing muscles- Muscles that work in opposition to the ones you are training. For example, the bicep is the opposing muscle to the triceps; the hamstring is the opposing muscle to the quadriceps.

Osteoporosis- A disease characterized by low bone mass and deterioration of bone tissue, which increases the risk of fracture.

Overload Principle- This principle says that to train muscles, they must work harder than they are accustomed to. This "overload" will result in increased strength as the body adapts to the stress placed upon it.

Overuse Injuries- Injuries that result from the cumulative effects of repetitive (day-after-day) stresses placed on tendons, muscles, and joints.

Percent grade- Measure of the elevation of a treadmill.

Physical fitness- The ability to perform regular to vigorous physical activity without great fatigue.

Pilates- Exercise programs that combine dynamic stretching with movement against resistance.

Plateau- Point in an exercise program where no additional progress is being made (gains in strength, weight loss, increased endurance, etc.). One way to break through a plateau is to change the kind of activity you are doing or something about your current activity- adding hills, increasing speed, increasing distance, etc.

247

PNF stretching- Proprioceptive neuromuscular facilitation (PNF) stretching is a static stretch of a muscle immediately after maximally contracting it.

Primary prevention- Actions designed to stop problems before they start.

Pronation- To turn or rotate (the foot) so that the inner edge of the sole bears the body's weight.

Plyometric training- Exercises that enable a muscle to reach maximal force production in as short a time as possible. For example, jumping from a 3 ft. stool to the ground and immediately springing back up to another stool.

Rate of perceived exertion (RPE)- Scale of 1-10 that rates how you are feeling (both physically and mentally) as it relates to exercise fatigue.

Repetition- The number of times an exercise is repeated within a single exercise "set."
Resistance training- See "Strength training"

Resting HR- Rate at which your heart beats at rest (while sitting or being inactive). Low resting heart rates are a good measure of health and fitness.

Resting Metabolic Rate (RMR)- Number of calories expended to maintain the body during resting conditions. Also referred to as basal metabolic rate.

Set- A basic unit of a workout containing the number of times (repetitions) a specific exercise is done (e.g., do 3 sets of 5 repetitions with 100 pounds).

Shin splint- Generic term used to describe pain in the lower leg, either on the medial (inside) or lateral side (outside) of the shin bone.

Sit and reach test- A common fitness test that decides flexibility (of the hamstrings and lower back).

Skinfold caliper test- A method of figuring out body fat whereby folds of skin and fat at various points on the body are grasped between thumb and forefinger and measured with calipers.

Skin fold measurements- This method of measuring body composition assumes that substantial fat is proportional to overall body fat, and thus by measuring several sites, total body fat may be calculated.

Slow twitch muscle fibers- Fibers that are better-suited for low-force, long duration activities because they have more endurance enzymes.

Specificity of Training Principle- This principle says that only the muscle or muscle group you exercise will respond to the demands placed upon it. By regularly doing curls, for example, the muscles involved (biceps) will become larger and stronger, but curls will have no effect on the muscles that are not being trained. Therefore, when strength training, it is important to strengthen all the major muscles.

Static stretching- A low force, high-duration stretch where the muscle is held at the greatest possible length for up to 30 seconds.

Strength training (resistance training)- The process of exercising with progressively heavier resistance for the purpose of strengthening the musculoskeletal system.

Systolic blood pressure- The pressure exerted on the vessel walls during ventricular

251

contraction, measured in millimeters of mercury. The systolic number is the top of the fraction. 120/80 is an average value for normal blood pressure (120 is the systolic number). Mild high blood pressure is considered to be between 140/90 and 160/95. High blood pressure is defined by a value greater than 160/95.

Tai chi- An ancient Chinese form of exercise, widely practiced in the West today, that promotes balance, coordination, stretching, and meditation.

Talk test- Method to ensure you are working out at a level where you can answer a question but not comfortably carry on a conversation. This is a good intensity level for weight loss and improved physical fitness.

Tapering- The process athletes use to reduce their training load for several days prior to competition.

Target heart rate (THR)- The recommended range is 60-85% of your maximum heart rate. It stands for a pace that ensures you are training aerobically and can reasonably be maintained.

Tension Principle- This principle says that tension is created by resistance, which can come from weights, bands, machines, or body weight.

Testosterone- The steroid hormone produced in the testes; involved in growth and development of muscle mass. Since men have more testosterone than women, they are able to gain muscle mass more easily.

Thyroid- Endocrine gland found in the neck that secretes T3 and T4 (hormones), which increase metabolic rate.

Type I muscle fibers- Fibers that hold large numbers of oxidative enzymes and are highly fatigue resistant (more prevalent in endurance athletes).

Type IIA muscle fibers- Fibers that hold biochemical and fatigue characteristics that are between Type IIB and Type I fibers (the best of both worlds).

Type IIB muscle fibers- Fibers that have a relatively small number of mitochondria, a limited capacity for aerobic metabolism, and are less resistant to fatigue than slow fibers (more prevalent in sprinters and power lifters).

Variable resistance- Strength training exercises that change the amount of resistance throughout the full range of motion.

Vigorous intensity- Activities above 60% of max heart rate. These activities cause an increased rate of breathing, sweating, and feel somewhat hard to hard.

Waist to hip ratio- A calculation of the proportion of fat stored on your body around your waist and hips. Formula: waist measurement divided by hip measurement. Women should have a ratio of 0.8 or less; men should have a ratio of .95 or less.

Warm up- To prepare for an athletic event (whether a game or a workout session) by exercising, stretching, or practicing for a brief time beforehand.

Yoga- A variety of Indian traditions geared toward self-discipline and the realization of unity; includes forms of exercise widely practiced in the West today that promote balance, coordination, flexibility, and meditation.

www.ingramcontent.com/pod-product-compliance
Lightning Source LLC
Chambersburg PA
CBHW051716020426
42333CB00014B/1008